Lectin Free Diet

The Cookbook with 75 Delicious
Lectin Free Meals to Aid Weight
Loss, Inhibit Inflammation and Other
Diseases

NATHAN MALLORY

ISBN: 9781728934518

DEDICATION

To my beloved mother, Rachael

TABLE OF CONTENTS

INTRODUCTION

As we all know, proteins are essential food nutrients that help build up the body cells. But not all proteins are beneficial; there are certain kinds of protein that can be potentially destructive to the body called lectins. They are known to possess certain properties that cause the dysfunction of the body systems such as the immune system, digestive system and other key metabolic activities. One of the ways these controversial proteins get into the body is through our diet. Studies have shown that eating a diet that is devoid of lectin containing foods will greatly reduce inflammation, help you lose weight and prevents other diseases.

What Are Lectins?

Lectins are sugar-binding proteins that have the ability to bind to cell membranes. They attach themselves to specific carbohydrate or glycoprotein molecules. They are naturally occurring proteins that can be found mainly in legumes, grains, seeds and nightshade vegetables. Lectins can cause interaction between cells without the interference of the immune system as they stick with other molecules in the cell membrane.

Lectins are primarily found in plants but they are also found in animals who feed majorly on grains. In plants, lectins are mainly found in grains, legumes and the cotyledon which is the portion of the plant seed that grows into the leaves. They act as a form of defense against predators like insects, microorganisms and pests; no wonder they cause a lot of pain and discomfort in humans when consumed in considerable amounts. When eaten by animals, the lectins in seeds help prevent them from being digested, thereby preserving the seeds for dispersal when excreted.

Harmful Effects of Lectins

1. **They damage the gut lining cells:** When lectins bind to the lining of the gastrointestinal tract, they hinder its repair and thereby causing the gut to "leak". Leaking gut is a condition whereby the intestinal lining loses its constraining ability and allows both the good and the unwanted substances to pass through to the blood, exposing the immune system to inflammatory agents (antigens).

2. **They stimulate the body immune system:** When these antigens get into the blood, they may trigger a wider immune response as the body produces antibodies and tries to attack the unfamiliar substances that have escaped through the gut wall in defense.

3. **They hinder absorption of nutrients:** Lectins also hinder the proper absorption of some vitamins and minerals by the intestinal walls and are sometimes referred to as antinutrients.

4. **They can cause inflammation:** A diet with a lot of lectins can cause inflammation, which is associated with arthritis, heart disease, Parkinson's disease and dementia.

5. **They are mostly indigestible:** Dietary lectins are mostly resistant to digestion and are excreted intact in feces. They can pass directly into the blood stream causing adverse immune response, obesity, autoimmunity and other harmful health conditions.

6. **They can cause weight gain:** Foods containing lectin like wheat can cause the body to store fat. Lectins mimic certain compounds in the body

called leptins which are responsible for controlling appetite or food satisfaction. They bind to the leptin receptors giving a wrong signal of hunger and therefore increasing calorie intake.

7. **They adversely affect the red blood cells:** by making them to clump together.

Since lectins can't be digested, the human body produces antibodies to dietary lectins. However, everyone has a different response to some particular lectins when consumed. Some lectins, like those found in red kidney beans called phytohaemagglutinin should be totally avoided as they can lead to poisoning.

Consumption of uncooked grains and legumes can lead to vomiting, nausea and diarrhea. Food high in lectin can also cause flatulence and lectin poisoning.

Reducing or Deactivating Lectin Content of Food

Sprouting- In some beans, seeds and grains, the lectins are found in the seed coat. By sprouting, these lectins are eliminated as the grains begin to germinate and the seed coat is metabolized.

Soaking and Cooking- This is probably the oldest and most widely practiced way of preparing grains and beans to reduce their lectin content. This is done by soaking the grains and beans overnight and changing the water at long intervals. Sometimes baking soda (or sodium bicarbonate) is added while soaking to augment the process. The grain and beans are then rinsed thoroughly for the last time and cooked by boiling for a few hours.

Fermenting- This is the process of breaking down carbohydrates or harmful substances by micro organisms like yeast and beneficial bacteria. If you've had beer, sourdough bread or soy beans products like tamari and tempeh, you've consumed fermented grains.

Pressure Cooking: This can also help in destroying lectins in foods like sweet potatoes, beans and squashes.

Peeling and Deseeding: The skin and seeds of some fruits and vegetables need to be removed before they are eaten. This is because these parts contain higher levels of lectin e.g. tomatoes and peppers. In the same way, the lectin rich skin (hull) of brown rice is removed in the process of making white rice, reducing the lectin content of the later.

So if you must eat legumes, grains or any lectin rich food, ensure you use one or two of the above methods to reduce or eliminate their lectin content.

Lectin Rich Foods

Here are some foods that have high lectin content. It will do you much good to stay away from these foods especially if you are sensitive to lectin.

Legumes- beans, peanuts, soy, cashew, peas and lentils

Nightshade vegetables- peppers, tomatoes, eggplant and potatoes

Grains- all types of grains

Dairy - milk (especially A1), cheese, yogurt

Gluten foods- malt, wheat, barley, rye and sometimes oats

Yeast- all yeast except nutritional yeast and brewer yeast

Foods to Eat In a Lectin Free Diet

There are still a variety of foods to choose from that are safe from lectins and their harmful effects. So, you can still enjoy a healthy balanced meal while following a lectin free diet. Below are different food groups and the various foods that you can eat freely in this diet.

Proteins

Beef

Fish

Chicken

Hemp protein

Pork

Bone broth

Eggs

Liver

A2 milk

Nuts and seeds- pistachios, hemp seeds, flax seeds, pecans, macadamia

Note: All animals that produce meat must be pasture raised (grass fed) and not grain fed.

Carbohydrates

Raw honey

Fruits- avocados, all berries

Starch- Japanese or purple sweet potatoes

Fats and Oils

Extra virgin olive oil

Caprylic acid

Avocados and avocado oil

Red palm oil

Ghee

Black cumin seed oil

Hemp seeds

Coconut and coconut oil

MCT oil

Macadamia oil

Organic sour and heavy cream

Vegetables

Celery

Romaine lettuce

Sprouts e.g. broccoli

Cucumber

Garlic and onion

Condiments and Sweeteners

Stevia

Mustard

Dulse powder

Xylitol

Nutritional yeast

Italian seasoning

Monk fruit

erythritol

Note: You can take in potassium and calcium supplement to fill in for the absence of dairy and other plant based foods.

Now that you are fully equipped with all there is to know about lectins and the kind of food you should stock your pantry with, you are ready to delve into the following chapters and enjoy healthy and delicious lectin free meals. The meals are categorised into breakfast, desserts and snacks, vegetarian, stews and soups, beef and pork, chicken and seafood. Just follow everything learnt in this book and you'll find out that following a lectin free diet plan is not a difficult exercise at all.

BREAKFAST RECIPES

Cassava Taco Cups

Preparation time: 30 minutes

Cooking time: 15 minutes

Servings: 12 taco cups

Ingredients:

1 cup cassava flour

Avocado oil, for greasing pan

¼ cup palm shortening or salted butter, melted

½ cup coconut milk, unsweetened, at room temperature

¼ cup water, warm

Directions:

1. Preheat the oven to 425°F. Grease the sides and bottom of a 12-cup muffin tin.

2. In a medium bowl, mix cassava flour, butter, coconut milk and warm water together until properly mixed. Divide the dough into 12 one-ounce balls.

3. With a pin or tortilla press, roll the dough balls between 2 pieces of parchment paper into small 4" rounds.

4. Peel the rolled dough from the parchment paper then spread over the undersides of muffin tins. Fold and press in the dough to stick to the shape of the cups.

5. Bake for about 20 minutes until golden brown then allow it cool before adding preferred toppings. Serve.

Storage tip: The cups/tins can be sealed then stored for up to 1 week at room temperature or freeze for up to 1 month. When ready to eat, bake for 8 to 10 minutes at 425°F. The taco cups will be crispier than previous cups.

Note: add ½ tsp of salt if the butter is not salted

Nutritional Information: Calories: 94; Total Fat: 4g; Total Carbs: 10g; Protein: 0.5g

No-Lectin Pancakes

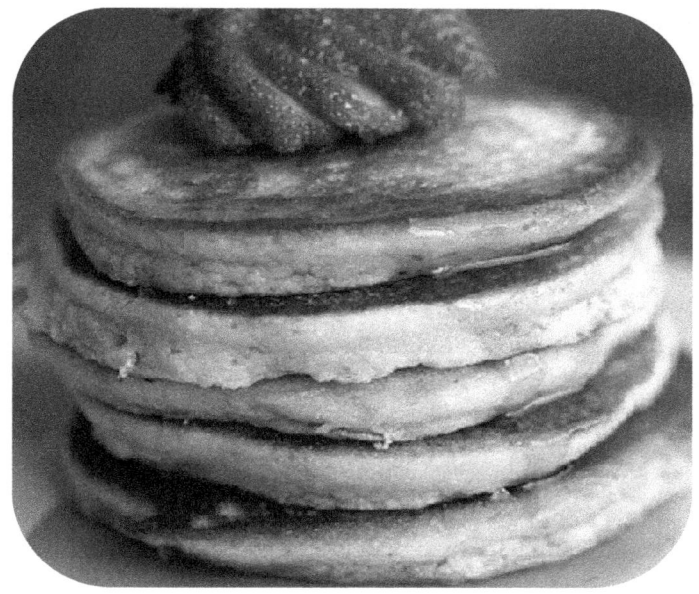

Enjoy a crispy lectin-free pancake topped with roasted vanilla bean sauce. Yummy!!

Preparation time: 15 minutes

Cooking time: 15 minutes

Servings: 4

Ingredients:

1 tablespoon baking powder

1 tablespoon melted coconut oil

¾ cup tapioca flour

1 cup almond flour

¼ teaspoon sea salt

2/3 cup almond milk, unsweetened

1 tablespoon maple syrup

2 teaspoons apple cider vinegar

1 teaspoon pure vanilla extract

Directions:

1. Blend all the ingredients in a blender, blending for some seconds then pause and scrape down the sides; blend for extra seconds.

2. Add small increments about ½ tbsp of flour or liquid if required in order to get a pancake batter texture.

3. Scoop about ¼ cup of batter for each pancake on oiled skillet over medium to medium-high heat.

4. Once a spatula slides under pancake with ease or the pancakes start to bubble, flip them over and continue cooking on both sides until golden brown.

5. Once done, let the pancakes slightly cool then serve.

6. Add toppings such as nut butter and roasted strawberry vanilla bean sauce.

Note: You may mix all the ingredients in a bowl to make the batter but blending the ingredients makes it fluffier.

Nutritional Information: Calories: 283; Total Fat: 18g; Total Carbs: 29g; Protein: 6g

Cheesy Cinnamon Pancake

Preparation time: 35 minutes

Cooking time: 35 minutes

Servings: 4

Ingredients:

1¼ cups goat's milk kefir, at room temperature (or almond/coconut yoghurt)

1 cup cassava flour

2 tbsp monk fruit sweetener

¼ tsp sea salt

1 tbsp baking powder

½ tsp vanilla extract

1 tsp cinnamon + extra for serving

2 large eggs, room temperature

1/8 tsp nutmeg

3 tbsp butter, melted or extra for serving

¼ cup water

Directions:

1. Preheat a nonstick griddle to medium-low heat.

2. In a medium bowl, combine beat the flour, baking powder, nutmeg, sweetener, sea salt and cinnamon together until well mixed.

3. In a large bowl, beat the kefir, eggs, water and vanilla together until well incorporated then whisk in butter.

4. In a large bowl, whisk the dry and wet mixture together until smooth and well mixed.

5. Pour batter on the heated griddle with a ¼ cup of measuring cup, pouring one to three pancakes at a time.

6. Cook for about 2 minutes until the top bubbles and the undersides are golden brown. With a spatula, flip the pancakes over and cook for another 1 minute.

7. Repeat the cooking process with the rest of the batter.

5. Serve at once or transfer the pancakes to a warm oven then cover with a towel slightly damp to keep them warm. Top with a sprinkle of cinnamon then serve with butter.

Nutritional Information: Calories: 242kcal; Total Fat: 11.78g; Total carbs: 29.46g; Protein: 4.71 g

Cheesy Spinach-Egg Breakfast Burritos

Preparation time: 10 minutes

Cooking time: 5 minutes

Servings: 4

Ingredients:

8 cassava flour tortillas (6 to 8")

4 oz crumbled goat cheese

2 tbsp extra-virgin olive oil

2 oz spinach, sliced

6 eggs, whisked

2 garlic cloves, sliced thin

Black pepper

Himalayan sea salt

Directions:

1. Pour oil into a large skillet then heat over medium heat.

2. Pour in the garlic, spinach, ½ teaspoon of pepper and salt then cook for 2 to 3 minutes until the spinach wilts.

3. Ladle the mixture equally across the pan then pour the whisked eggs on top. Let it sit for about 30 seconds. Using a spatula, move the eggs around the pan for 3 to 4 minutes until set.

4. Turn the heat off then spread the goat cheese over the eggs then let it soften.

5. On the other hand, cover the tortillas with a damp paper towel then heat up in the microwave. Heat up about 4 at a time for 30 seconds.

6. Scoop the eggs into the middle of each tortilla then fold like taco. Serve.

Nutritional Information: Calories: 531kcal; Fat: 23.69g; Carbs: 50.15g; Protein 27.18 g

Almond Breakfast Biscuits

Whip up an easy and lectin free breakfast of almond flour biscuits with a hearty stew topped with cream and berries.

Preparation time: 5 minutes

Cooking time: 20 minutes

Servings: 4

Ingredients:

1 teaspoon baking powder

1½ cup almond flour, blanched (don't use almond meal)

3 tablespoon coconut or heavy cream

½ teaspoon kosher salt

3 tablespoons cold butter, chopped small

1 egg

Directions:

1. Preheat the oven to 350°F.

2. Line a cookie sheet with parchment paper then set it aside.

3. Combine baking powder, flour and salt in a medium-sized bowl.

4. Add the chopped butter, using a butter knife or pastry cutter to cut the butter into the flour.

5. Continue cutting the butter into smaller sizes while pressing into the flour until all the chunky ones disappear and the dough becomes crumbly.

6. Create a well in the center of the bowl then crack in one egg. Add the cream then lightly blend the cream and egg together with a fork. Now, slowly mix with the dough until it incorporates and soft dough forms.

7. Divide the dough into four sizes with your hands then roll into balls. The dough should be soft and slightly sticky.

8. Set the dough balls on the lined cookie sheet, make sure the dough isn't flattened.

9. Now bake for 20 minutes until a bit golden. Allow it cool a bit then slice.

10. Top with delicious jam or whipped cream/coconut cream and berries.

Nutritional Information: Calories: 148kcal; Fat: 15.17g; Carbs: 1.11g; Protein 2.84g

Healthy Greenie Smoothie

Preparation time: 5 minutes

Cooking time: 0 minute

Servings: 1

Ingredients:

½ cup desired greens (chard, kale, spinach)

½ avocado, ripe

½ cup coconut milk, or water

1 ripe banana

1 cup ice

Directions:

1. In a blender, pulse the banana, avocado and ice then top with desired greens.

2. Process until smooth then add more water or coconut milk if it isn't blending well.

Nutritional Information: Calories: 588kcal; Fat: 44.51g; Carbs: 49.43g; Protein: 11.76

No-Lectin Tapioca Pasta

Whip up a quick lectin free breakfast of tapioca pasta with just four simple ingredients.

Preparation time: 10 minutes

Cooking time: 10 minutes

Servings: 4

Ingredients:

1 cup tapioca starch/flour, + more for dusting

2 large eggs

1 cup super fine almond flour

Olive oil

1 teaspoon kosher salt

Directions:

1. In a bowl, combine almond and tapioca flour.

2. Create a space in center of the flour mixture then break in the eggs. Using a fork, stir the eggs then whisk your way out, mixing in more of the flour.

3. When the egg is well mixed with the flour, use your hands to knead the mixture, pouring a little more tapioca flour if the dough is sticky. Separate dough into 3 sizes.

4. Cover the cutting board and rolling pin with tapioca flour. Take one of the dough portions then dust lightly before you roll it out into about 1/8" thickness.

5. Cut the rolled out dough with a pizza cutter into desired thickness of noodles then scoop up the noodles with a large spatula so they don't break.

6. Boil 4 qt of water in a large pot then add 1 tbsp of olive oil. Once it starts to boil, add the noodles then cook for 2 minutes.

7. Use a slotted spoon to take out the noodles from water then transfer to a pasta strainer.

8. Sprinkle olive oil on top so they don't stick together. Repeat this cooking process with rest of the dough.

Note: Don't use almond meal, make sure you use super fine almond flour.

Nutritional Information: Calories: 593kcal; Fat: 14.5g; Carbs: 105.4g; Protein 8.2g

Cheesy Spinach Breakfast Omelet

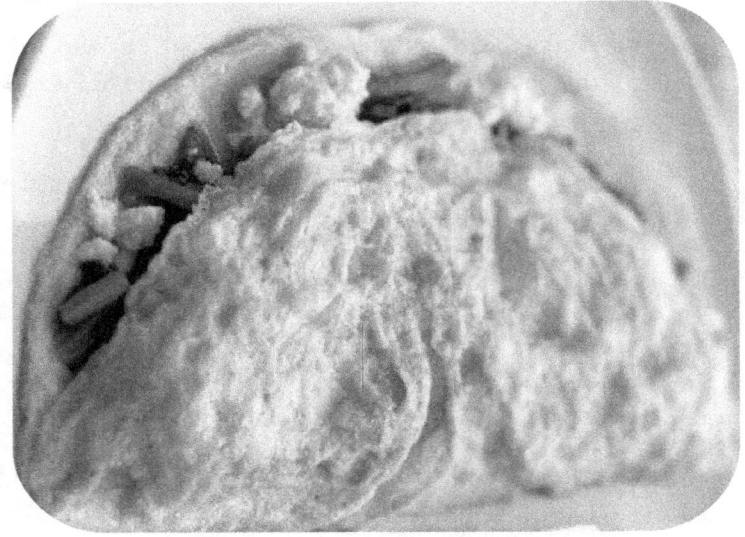

Preparation time: 5 minutes

Cooking time: 6 minutes

Servings: 1

Ingredients:

1 cup frozen spinach or 2 cups freshly chopped

1 tablespoon butter, divided

1 cup chopped parsley

1 tablespoon feta cheese

¼ cup finely diced scallions or white onion

½ teaspoon dried thyme

1 garlic clove, finely chopped

2 eggs

½ teaspoon dried oregano

Pepper to taste

Salt to taste

Optional: 1 cup arugula, dressed in 1 tsp of olive oil

Directions:

1. To make the spinach filling; melt ½ tbsp of butter over medium-high heat then add the onion and garlic, stirring until translucent and aromatic.

2. Add the spinach, oregano, parsley and thyme. Continue cooking for about 3 to 4 minutes until most of the liquid from parsley and spinach evaporate. Add pepper and salt to taste. Note that some feta cheese brands can be salty.

3. Transfer the spinach filling to a bowl then set aside.

4. To prepare the omelet; In a bowl, crack in 2 eggs, add pepper and a pinch of salt then whisk the eggs.

5. Melt the rest of the butter in the pan over medium high heat. Pour in the eggs, swirling the pan and pushing the edges with a rubber spatula so the egg continues to cook.

6. Once the omelet is almost done, flip over.

7. Top egg with spinach filling then sprinkle one tbsp of feta cheese on top. Fold and keep cooking until the egg is ready.

Nutritional Information: Calories: 349kcal; Total Fat: 28g; Total Carb: 11.5g;

Protein: 17.3g

Savory Sweet Potato Scallion Hash

Enjoy a well spiced lectin-free breakfast of sweet potatoes with scrambled eggs and poblano pepper topped with scallions.

Preparation time: 10 minutes

Cooking time: 40 minutes

Servings: 2 - 4

Ingredients:

2 medium peeled sweet potatoes, chopped into small cubes

1 teaspoon smoked paprika

2 tablespoon avocado/olive oil

½ teaspoon turmeric

¼ - ½ teaspoon ground black pepper

½ teaspoon sea salt

1 poblano pepper, deseed then diced (optional)

½ teaspoon powdered onion

Scallions, sliced on the bias (only the green parts)

2 garlic cloves, finely chopped

Directions:

1. Heat up oven to 400°F.

2. Toss the sweet potato cubes with oil in a medium or large bowl then add turmeric, paprika, black pepper, sea salt and powdered onion. Mix until well combined.

3. Pour mixture onto a sheet pan. Split the sweet potatoes among two pans if the pan is crowded, so that you don't get steamed potatoes at the end.

4. Bake for 20 minutes then take out the pan from the oven. Stir the sweet potatoes gently so you don't smash them.

5. Add the diced pepper then return to the oven for extra 10 to 15 minutes.

6. During the last 5 minutes of cooking time, take out the pan again then add the finely chopped garlic cloves.

7. If the potatoes are turning very dark, you can turn off the oven and allow the potatoes cook with the residual heat. You may leave the oven door open to let some heat escape. The garlic should barely cook.

8. Take out from the oven then top with scallions. Serve at once with tofu scramble or scrambled eggs, hot sauce or tempeh bacon if desired.

Note: Leave out the pepper, if you are strictly lectin-free.

Nutritional Information: Calories: 173kcal; Total Fat: 9.33g; Total Carb: 21.67g; Protein 2.15 g

Lectin-Free Tempeh Bacon

Preparation time: 5 minutes

Cooking time: 5 minutes

Servings: 2 - 4

Ingredients:

8 oz. tempeh, grain-free and sliced thin

2 tablespoons coconut oil

¼ teaspoon ground black pepper

3 tablespoon coconut aminos

1 tablespoon olive oil

¼ teaspoon sea salt

1 tablespoon rice wine vinegar

1 teaspoon smoked paprika

¼ teaspoon liquid smoke

5 drops liquid stevia

Pinch of cayenne, optional

Directions:

1. In a shallow dish, combine all the ingredients, except coconut oil and tempeh.

2. Add the slices of tempeh then flip until well coated. Let it marinate for 5 minutes.

3. On the other hand, heat up pan to medium-high; add 1 tbsp of coconut oil.

4. After marinating, turn down the heat to medium then add the slices of tempeh, ensuring the pan isn't crowded. Cook in few batches.

5. Cook for 2 to 4 minutes, flipping from time to time until both sides are brown. Take note that they burn easily, so stay close.

6. Pour coconut oil into the pan if necessary. If there is still marinade in the pan, turn down the heat to medium-low towards the end of cooking time then scoop the marinade over the slices while they cook. Do thus carefully because the liquid is hot and might splatter.

Nutritional Information: Calories: 400kcal; Total Fat: 35.13g; Total Carb: 17.27g; Protein: 5.73 g

Sweetened Millet Granola

Enjoy a grain free breakfast granola made with millet seeds and sweetened with dates and honey. Yummy!!!

Preparation time: 5 minutes

Cooking time: 30 minutes

Servings: 6

Ingredients:

½ cup raw millet, cooked according to directions on the package

1 cup shredded coconut

½ cup dates

2 teaspoons cinnamon, divided

¼ cup of melted coconut oil

1 teaspoon vanilla extract

¼ cup of almond butter

1 cup pecans, diced coarsely

1 tablespoon honey (maple syrup or agave) optional

1 cup walnuts, diced coarsely

Optional: 1 tablespoon ground flaxseed, 2 tablespoon almond flour

¼ cup water

Pinch of salt

Directions:

1. Heat up oven to 300°F. Line 1 or 2 baking sheets with parchment paper.

2. Combine coconut, honey, dates, coconut oil, vanilla extract, 1 teaspoon of cinnamon almond butter and water in a food processor until you get a sticky paste. It's alright if some chunks are still visible.

3. In a large bowl, combine cooked millet, walnuts, pecans and the optional ingredients if desired.

4. Pour the date mixture into the bowl then mix everything together properly.

5. Add the remaining 1 teaspoon of cinnamon and a pinch of salt on top.

6. Once it's properly mixed, spread the granola onto the prepared baking sheet.

7. Bake for 20 minutes in the top or middle rack of the oven. Once done, take out from the oven then stir.

8. Return to the oven and bake for another 35 to 40 minutes. Take it out every 10 minutes and stir.

9. Turn down the heat of the oven to 275°F, if any of the pieces are turning too dark and watch it closely.

10. Once done, take out from the oven then let it completely cool for storing in an airtight container for up to five days in a cupboard. You may let it cool overnight on top of the oven so it dries completely and becomes crispier.

Notes: 10 to 11 dates were used and dried out.

Nutritional Information: Calories: 582kcal; Total Fat: 46.9g; Total Carb: 36.4g; Protein: 12.3g

CHICKEN RECIPES

Mandarin Sauced Chicken Meatballs

Prepare a hearty dinner of grain free chicken meatballs in mandarin orange sauce, suitable for the whole family.

Preparation time: 10 minutes

Cooking time: 30 minutes

Servings: 4 (18 meatballs)

Ingredients:

For the Mandarin Orange Sauce:

2 tablespoons coconut aminos/liquid aminos/tamari or soy sauce

1 teaspoon avocado oil

2 garlic cloves, minced finely

1 tablespoon ginger root, chopped finely

½ teaspoon Sriracha

1 teaspoon sesame oil

½ cup chicken stock

1 tablespoon orange zest

¼ cup mandarin orange juice, freshly squeezed

1 teaspoon tapioca starch

1 teaspoon honey, optional

For the chicken meatballs:

1 lb ground chicken (don't use ground chicken breast)

1 tablespoon orange zest

¼ cup almond flour

2 garlic cloves, minced finely

1 teaspoon coconut aminos/liquid aminos/tamari or soy sauce

¼ cup scallions, sliced finely

1 tablespoon ginger root, chopped finely

½ teaspoon sesame oil

1 teaspoon avocado oil

3 large mushrooms, dice finely (or 1 cup if finely chopped)

Kosher salt

For garnish: Extra scallions and sesame seeds

Directions:

1. To prepare the meatballs; preheat the oven to 400°F. Heat oil in a pan over medium high heat then add ginger and garlic then sauté for 1 minute until aromatic.

2. Pour in the scallions and mushrooms then season with a pinch of salt. Stir for about 3 minutes until mushrooms release their liquid. Remove from heat then cool a bit.

3. Combine chicken, orange zest, coconut aminos, sesame oil and almond flour in a large bowl then add the sautéed vegetables. Mix everything together with a wooden spoon.

4. Damp your hands then mold mixture into balls. You can use a tablespoon measure so come out the same size and note that the mixture will be very soft.

5. Set the balls on a baking sheet line with parchment then bake for 20 minutes.

6. Meanwhile, prepare the sauce. Heat up a pan over medium high heat then add 1 teaspoon of avocado oil then add garlic and ginger.

7. Combine the rest of the ingredients except garnishing ingredients in a small bowl. Now pour this into the heated pan. Stir while cooking for 3 minutes until the sauce thickens a bit.

8. Immediately the meatballs are ready, add them to the sauce then stir gently to coat.

Top with sesame seeds and extra scallions of desired. Note that the sauce will be thick. You can also serve over cauli-rice or steamed broccoli

Nutritional Information: Calories: 259kcal; Total Fat: 15.4g; Total Carb: 9.3g;

Protein: 21.7g

Veggie-Chicken LoMein

Prepare this inspiring dish of noodle packed with veggies and chicken. Tastes real good.

Preparation time: 15 minutes

Cooking time: 15 minutes

Servings: 4

Ingredients:

For the noodles:

8 oz. shirataki noodles, spaghetti type (2 packages)

2 - 3 cups slaw mix (a mix of carrots, green and red cabbage)

2 teaspoon avocado oil

4 garlic cloves, finely diced

½ tablespoon ginger, minced

2 chicken breasts, sliced into small chunks

1 tablespoon sesame seeds, optional

1 tablespoon scallions, optional

1 cup white onion slices (or 1 small onion)

For the sauce:

½ teaspoon arrowroot or tapioca starch

3 tablespoon coconut aminos/soy sauce/tamari

½ teaspoon sriracha

2 teaspoons rice vinegar

1 teaspoon sesame oil

2 tablespoons water

1 teaspoon honey (optional)

Directions:

1. To make the noodles; soak the shirataki noodles in water for about 2 to 3 minutes then drain liquid in a colander and give a final rinse.

2. Transfer the drained noodles to a pan placed over medium-high heat. Stir the noodles for about 4 minutes until it dries completely then set aside.

3. To make the sauce, in a small bowl, combine all the sauce ingredients then whisk until well mixed. Set aside.

4. Heat two teaspoons of avocado oil in a pan over medium-high heat then add the minced ginger and garlic. Sauté for about 30 minutes until aromatic.

5. Add the chicken chunks then stir everything together. Keep cooking until chicken is well cooked and browned. Deglaze the pan with one tablespoon of the prepared sauce, ensuring all the bits stuck to the pan are scraped up. Set the chicken aside once it is coated and the pan has been deglazed.

6. Using the same pan without giving it a rinse, pour in onion slices then cook for 2 minutes until it begins to soften. Pour in the slaw mixture then stir until the juices release and the cabbage begins to soften.

7. For a crunchy slaw, sauté for some minutes. Keep stirring for a tender veggie.

8. Add the prepared noodles and the cooked chicken. Pour in the rest of the sauce then mix everything together with tongs so the noodles are covered with sauce. Heat through.

9. Serve chicken and veggie lo-mein on a dish then garnish with scallions and sesame seeds.

Nutritional Information: Calories: 163kcal; Total Fat: 3.9g; Total Carb: 13.1g; Protein: 12.6g

Cheesy Mushroom 'N' Chicken Enchiladas

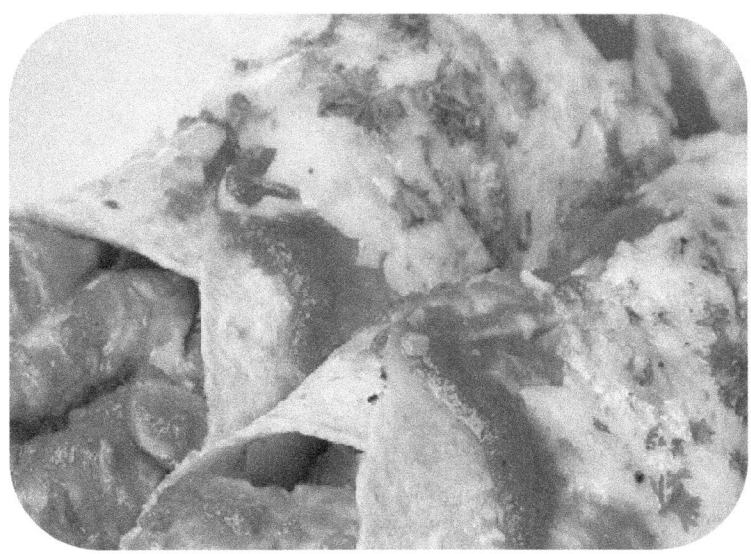

Preparation time: 30 minutes

Cooking time: 15 minutes

Servings: 8 enchiladas

Ingredients:

8 oz. shiitake mushrooms, sliced

8 oz. shredded pastured chicken, cooked

8 oz. crumbled goat cheese

2 tbsp olive oil

4 peeled garlic cloves

1 white onion, diced

2 cup of broth, divided

3 tsp apple cider vinegar

Black pepper

Sea salt

1 tsp coconut aminos

½ tsp ground cumin

1 tsp granular sweetener

8 warmed cassava flour tortillas

¼ tsp paprika

½ tsp dried oregano

For serving: Hot sauce, chopped fresh cilantro

Directions:

1. Preheat the oven to 400°F.

2. In a large non-stick skillet, heat oil over medium-high heat. Add the onions and mushrooms then cook for 6 to 8 minutes, stirring from time to time until it starts to soften.

3. Pour in half cup of broth, the chicken, half teaspoon of salt and ¼ tsp of pepper. Lower heat to medium and cook, stirring frequently for 3 to 4 minutes, until most the liquid is absorbed.

4. Transfer this mixture to a large bowl then stir in half of the goat cheese.

5. To prepare the adobo sauce; combine garlic, the remaining broth, vinegar, paprika, oregano, coconut aminos, cumin, sweetener and 2 tsp of sea salt in a blender then pulse for about minutes until extremely smooth.

6. Pour the ½ cup of the sauce into a 9 by 13" glass baking dish. Scoop a dollop of the mushroom mixture into each tortilla then roll up. Place the rolled tortilla in the pan with seal side facing down.

7. Once the tortillas have been rolled and placed side-by-side in the pan, pour the rest of the adobo sauce on top then sprinkle the rest of the goat cheese on top.

8. Place in the oven then bake for 15 minutes until the sauce starts to bubble and the cheese has completely melted.

9. Sprinkle cilantro and hot sauce top. Serve.

Nutritional Information: Calories: 324kcal; Total Fat: 13.8g; Total Carb: 30.8g; Protein: 19.4g

Italian Chick'n Salad

Preparation time: 15 minutes

Cooking time: 0 minute

Servings: 2

Ingredients:

For the chicken salad

2 cups diced roasted chicken

½ head romaine lettuce

1 carrot, diced

½ cup jicama cubes

1 avocado, sliced

For the Italian Dressing

½ cup avocado oil

¼ cup fresh lemon juice

½ tsp black pepper (or to taste)

2 garlic cloves

1½ tsp sea salt (or to taste)

Directions:

1. To prepare the salad: Toss chicken, lettuce, avocado, preferred amount of dressing, jicama and carrot in a large bowl. Season with salt and pepper.

2. To prepare the dressing: In a blender, puree all the ingredients for sauce then season with salt and pepper to taste.

Nutritional Information: Calories: 850kcal; Total Fat: 73.1g; Total Carb: 25.1g; Protein: 29.6g

Garlicky Grilled Chicken

Preparation time: 12 minutes

Cooking time: 13 minutes

Servings: 4 - 6

Ingredients:

6 chicken thighs, skin on

6 cloves garlic, finely chopped

½ lemon, juice

Lemon wedges (optional)

1½ tsp sea salt

Directions:

1. To prepare the marinade; in a large mixing bowl, combine garlic, lemon juice and salt then stir. Set aside.

2. Use kitchen shears to take out bones from the chicken thighs. Transfer the bones into a zip-lock bag then freeze. Keep it for making chicken stock.

3. Set the chicken thigh on a cutting board with its skin side up. Cover them with a plastic wrap then pound with meat mallet using the flat side. Pound until the chicken is even, about ½" - ¾" thick.

4. Transfer the flattened chicken into the marinade then coat all over. Repeat this process with the rest of the chicken.

5. Heat up a cast iron griddle to medium heat.

6. Once it's hot, set the marinated chicken on the rack with its skin side down then grill for 8 minutes. Turn the chicken over with tongs then grill for another 5 minutes.

7. Once grilled, remove the chicken then allow it rest for 3 to 5 minutes.

8. Slice then serve with lemon wedges.

Nutritional Information: Calories: 115kcal; Total Fat: 3.6g; Total Carb: 3.6g; Protein: 16.9g

Crispy Chicken Nuggets

These lectin-free chicken nuggets are absolutely delicious, crispy and flavorful.

Preparation time: 10 minutes

Cooking time: 15 minutes

Servings: 4 - 6

Ingredients:

2 chicken breasts, sliced equally into 2"-3" long and ½" thick

2 eggs

2/3 cup of tapioca flour

2/3 cup of blanched almond flour

½ tsp onion granules

½ tsp paprika

1 tsp sea salt

½ cup of avocado oil

Directions:

1. Combine tapioca and almond flour, paprika, onion granules and salt in a big mixing bowl then whisk together. Ensure you remove any lumps from the almond flour.

2. Whisk the eggs and chicken slices together in a medium-sized mixing bowl, coat properly.

3. Dredge 3 to 4 coated chicken slices in the flour mixture then coat completely with breading.

4. Shake off excess breading then set the coated chicken on a parchment lined cookie sheet. Repeat this process with the rest of the chicken slices.

5. Heat up avocado oil in a medium-sized cast iron skillet over medium-low flame.

6. Once it's hot, add 4 to 5 chicken slices, ensuring the skillet isn't overcrowded. Cook each side for about 2 to 3 minutes until it turns golden brown.

7. Once done, transfer the chicken nuggets to a plate lined with paper towel. Repeat this process with the rest of the chicken slices.

8. Serve with barbeque sauce or ketchup.

Note: Chicken nuggets can be refrigerated in a ziplock bag for up to 3 days.

Nutritional Information: Calories: 152kcal; Total fat: 8.1g; Total Carb: 14.6g; Protein: 6.9g

Lemony Chick'n Salad Mixed with Avocado Berry Mayonnaise

Preparation time: 15 minutes

Cooking time: 30 minutes

Servings: 4 - 6

Ingredients:

2 chicken breasts, pasture raised

Lemon and Avocado oil

Lemon slices

Pepper

Salt

½ cup dry cranberries, unsweetened

2 - 3 stacks celery, diced finely

½ cup avocado mayonnaise

2 tbsp finely chopped tarragon (few stems of fresh tarragon)

Juice from ¼ lemon

Pepper

Salt to taste

Directions:

1. To make the chicken; preheat the oven to 370°F.

2. Place the chicken breasts in a pan then drizzle lemon and avocado oil on top then place few lemon slices on top. Sprinkle with pepper and salt.

3. Cover the pan with aluminum foil, don't touch the chicken then bake for 30 minutes.

4. Once done, remove from the oven then let it cool. Shred the chicken into small sizes or chop with a knife.

5. To make the salad; chop the tarragon, celery and tarragon finely. chop the cranberries into smaller pieces if they are too big.

6. Combine the chopped veggies and fruit with the shredded chicken then add mayonnaise, lemon juice, olive oil, pepper and salt, season to taste.

7. Store in an air tight glass container.

Nutritional Information: Calories: 433kcal; Total fat: 27.5g; Total carb: 28g; Protein: 21.6g

Rice 'N' Salad Chicken Rolls

Preparation time: 40 minutes

Cooking time: 15 minutes

Servings: 2

Ingredients:

For the rolls:

1 cup of chicken salad

1 pack organic rice

Baby arugula, few handfuls

3 Nori sheets, roasted

For serving:

Coconut aminos

Pickled ginger

Red radishes, sliced finely

Hot sauce

Wasabi paste

Directions:

1. Prepare the rice according to the directions on the pack. Once done, let i cool or refrigerate if cooked in advance.

2. Now, prepare the wasabi paste; mix 2 tablespoons of pure wasabi powde with enough cold water into a paste then set it aside.

3. Prepare the fillings then place the nori sheet on the bamboo sheet.

4. Fill the sheets with rice, then stack with the other fillings.

5. Roll, ensure you don't cover the whole sheet with filling.

6. Wet the upper edge of the rolls with cold water stick the two sides together. Continue with the second and third roll. Slice each rolls into 6 smaller ones.

7. Serve with coconut aminos, wasabi, pickled ginger, hot sauce and red radishes. **Nutritional Information:** Calories: 455kcal; Total fat: 2.9g; Total carb: 89.2g; Protein: 14.1g

Chicken Tenders

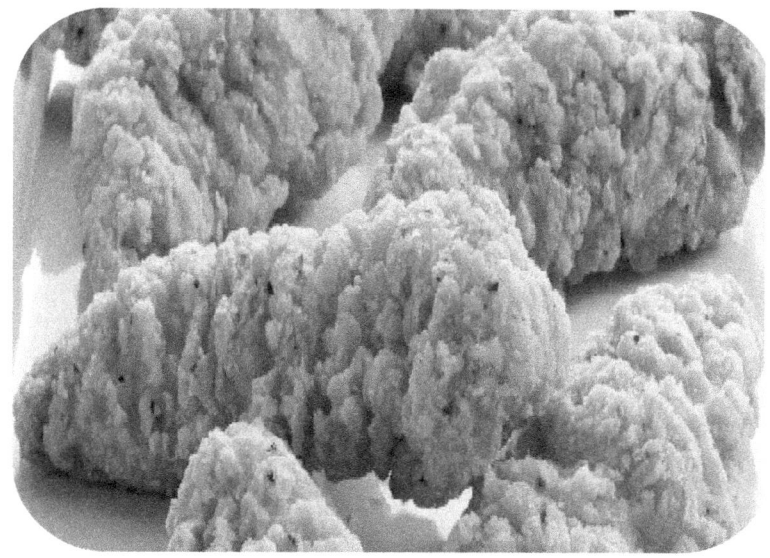

Preparation time: 25 minutes

Cooking time: 25 minutes

Servings: 4

Ingredients:

2 chicken breasts, halves, pasture raised

2/3 cup almond flour

2 eggs, pasture raised

½ cup cassava flour

Avocado oil

Spices:

Powdered onion

Hungarian paprika

Iodized sea salt

Organic garlic

Pepper

Directions:

1. Preheat oven to 400°F.

2. Slice chicken breasts into stripes lengthwise then sprinkle with the spices.

3. Pour cassava flour and almond flour into two separate bowls.

4. Whisk the eggs properly in a deep plate then add some pepper and salt.

5. Coat chicken slices with a thin layer of cassava flour then dredge each stripe in the whisked egg.

6. Now, coat with the almond flour.

7. Place the coated chicken stripes on an oven pan greased with avocado oil or lined parchment paper.

8. Bake for 15 to 20 minutes, baking time depends on how big the stripes are. Check after 15 minutes, so you don't overcook them.

Note: You can refrigerate in an air tight glass container for some days. They can be eaten cold or warm.

Nutritional Information: Calories: 325kcal; Total fat: 15.2g; Total carb: 15.5g; Protein: 31g

Noodles with Seaweed Chicken Salad

Preparation time: 15 minutes

Cooking time: 15 minutes

Servings: 2

Ingredients:

2 - 3 medium chicken nuggets, cooked (or few cooked chicken breast slices)

1 pack seaweed mixed sea vegetables, rinsed then re-salted according to directions

2 cups romaine lettuce

1 pack Noodles, angel hair, cooked according to directions

2 cups baby spinach

1 avocado, chopped

For the dressing:

4 tbsp coconut aminos

1 clove garlic, grated

4 tbsp apple cider vinegar

1 fresh ginger, thumb size and grated

Pepper

Salt to taste

Directions:

1. Cook the noodles according to the directions on the pack. Rinse, boil then dry. This should take about 15 minutes.

2. Prepare the seaweed according to the directions on the pack, rinse then allow to dry.

3. Prepare the dressing by mixing all the ingredients.

4. Wash then chop the romaine lettuce

5. Divide the noodles into two portions in two serving bowls.

6. Divide the remaining ingredients into two then add on the noodles.

7. Add the chicken breasts/slices.

8. Add the dressing, mix properly then taste. Add extra vinegar and aminos if required.

Nutritional Information: Calories: 675kcal; Total fat: 43.2g; Total carb: 152.3g; Protein: 27.1g

BEEF AND PORK RECIPES

Homemade Meatballs

Preparation time: 10 minutes

Cooking time: 7 minutes

Servings: 4 - 6

Ingredients:

1 pound ground beef, grass-fed

2 tsp ground flaxmeal

4 cloves garlic, minced finely

1 tsp coconut oil

1 whole egg

1 tsp sea salt

1/3 cup diced cilantro

Directions:

1. Combine beef, egg, flaxmeal, cilantro, garlic and salt in a large mixing bowl. Mix with a stand mixer or your hands until well mixed.

2. Scoop 1 tbsp of the beef mixture and mold into a ball, making about 23 meatballs.

3. Heat up coconut oil in a cast iron skillet over medium low heat. Once heated, add the meatballs and cook for about 5 to 7 minutes, turning from time to time so that all the sides are evenly browned. Cut the meatball in half to check if its properly cooked.

4. Serve with marinara and zucchini noodles.

Nutritional Information: Calories: 54kcal; Total fat: 3.4g; Total carb: 0.8g Protein: 4.1g

Baked Veggies 'N' Rhubarb Meatballs

Preparation time: 20 minutes

Cooking time: 40 minutes

Servings: Many

Ingredients:

1 lbs beef/ sirloin

2 eggs, pasture raised

1 bunch flat leaf parsley

5 medium button mushrooms

1 red onion, big

1 tablespoon cassava flour

2 big cloves garlic

1 bunch fresh basil leaves

Spices: dry oregano, salt (about 1 tsp) and pepper

2 cups rice cauliflower

2 - 3 tablespoons nutritional yeast

Extra virgin olive oil

2 cups broccoli slaw

1 cup diced rhubarb

Spices: Oregano and Herbs de Provence/Italian herbs

Pepper

Salt

Extra virgin olive oil

Directions:

1. Preheat the oven to 375°F.

2. Chop the parsley, basil, mushrooms, red onion and garlic in a food processor.

3. Transfer the chopped veggies to a mixing bowl then add the ground beef, cassava flour, 2 eggs, salt and spices. Mix properly with your hands.

4. Mold 1 tbsp of the beef mixture into balls.

5. Grease one big and two half sheet pans with olive oil.

6. Pour some cassava flour into a plate then roll the meatballs in the flour.

7. Now add the meatballs to the sheet pan. Repeat with the rest of the meatballs then drizzle olive oil on top.

8. Bake meatballs at 375°F for 20 minutes, flip them then bake for extra 5 minutes.

9. Remove meatballs from the pan. Without washing the pan, add the cauliflower rice, rhubarb and broccoli slaw to the pan.

10. Drizzle enough amounts of extra virgin olive oil on veggies then sprinkle with pepper, salt and the spices. Bake for about 15 minutes.

11. Take it out from the oven then serve with the meatballs, fresh veggies and hot sauce.

Nutritional Information: Calories: 215kcal; Total fat: 7.7g; Total carb: 14.2g; Protein: 24.4g

Herby Bourbon Beef Pate

Preparation time: 15 minutes

Cooking Time: 15 minutes

Servings: 8

Ingredients:

1 lbs beef liver, grass-fed

1 small red onion (or ½ of big one)

3 garlic cloves, crushed

Extra virgin olive oil

4 – 5 oz ghee

1 shot bourbon

3 tbsp of mixed fresh herbs (thyme, rosemary, sage) washed, dried and chopped

Pepper

Salt

Pinch of fresh grated nutmeg

Directions:

1. Take out the liver then pat dry and clean. Set aside on paper towels.

2. Prepare the herbs; washed, dried then chopped.

3. Chop the onion then crush the garlic and add them to a heated pan with generous amount of olive oil. Sauté for about 10 minutes until translucent and aromatic but not burnt. Remove content from the pan and set aside.

4. Spoon about 2 teaspoons of ghee into the pan then add the liver, heat to medium-high. Add the chopped herbs, pepper and salt.

5. Cook each side for 1 to 2 minutes then flip over and cook for another minute. Add a shot of bourbon (be careful if you have a flame).

6. Keep checking to see if they are cooked by slicing the middle with a knife and if it isn't pink in the middle. Ensure live don't overcook. Take them out once done and note that some might take a bit longer to cook due to their thickness.

7. In a blender or food process, add the liver, the contents from the pan, cooked garlic and onions, 2 tsp of ghee, pepper, grated nutmeg, salt and a few tbsp of olive oil. Pulse until you get a paste.

8. Taste and add season to your taste. You can add extra oil, pepper and salt if required.

9. Transfer to a non-plastic storage container or bowl with a lid. Level it up then top with a layer of ghee. Garnish with more herbs or extra pieces of cooked liver.

10. Refrigerate for up to 2 weeks.

Note: Don't overcook the liver. Reserve small amount of cooked liver for garnishing if desired. Topping with ghee isn't compulsory but it adds more flavour and it aids storage.

Nutritional Information: Calories: 188kcal; Total fat: 12.7g; Total carb: 3.9g; Protein: 11.8g

Hot Vegetable Packed Meatballs

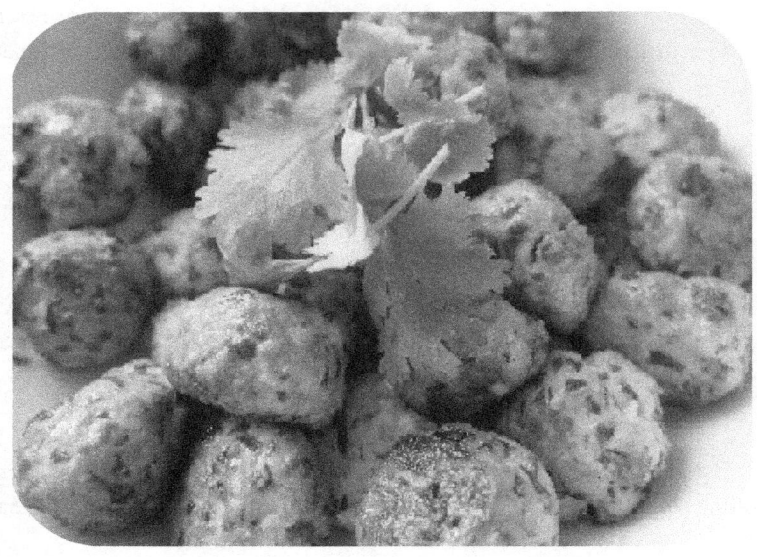

Preparation time: 50 minutes

Cooking time: 30 minutes

Servings: 6

Ingredients:

0.65 lbs ground beef, grass fed

2 tbsp Kimchi Sriracha Sauce, red (or additional for hot food)

½ cup fresh cilantro

8 oz baked mashed purple sweet potato

1 fresh ginger, thumb size and grated

3 scallions

1 fresh turmeric, thumb size and grated

1 - 2 stacks of celery

1 egg, pasture raised

2 cloves garlic cloves, grated

3 tbsp of cassava flour

Pepper

½ tsp iodized salt

Avocado oil plus toasted sesame seeds

For the vegetable bed:

2 cups cauliflower rice

2 – 3 tbsp coconut milk, full fat

2 cups broccoli slaw

2 – 3 tbsp avocado oil

1 tbsp rice vinegar

2-3 tbsp coconut aminos

Pepper

Salt to taste

Sesame seeds (optional)

1 tsp of arrowroot powder (optional)

Directions:

1. Preheat the oven to 400°F then grease a large sheet pan with a mixture of avocado oil and toasted sesame oil.

2. In a food processor, combine all the veggies properly to get a soft consistency or mix less to get a more chunky consistency.

3. Transfer the veggies to a large mixing bowl, add the egg, meat, pepper, salt, sauce and cassava flour.

4. Mold about 1 tablespoon of the mixture into meatball shape then set them on the oiled pan, creating little space in between.

5. Bake for 30 minutes at 400°F.

6. Serve with veggies or kimchi sriracha sauce. You can serve hot or cold.

7. To make the veggie bed; In a skillet, heat up avocado over medium heat.

8. Add the broccoli slaw and cauliflower rice then cook for 5 minutes.

9. Pour in the coconut milk, rice vinegar and coconut aminos then season with pepper and salt to taste and cook for some minutes.

10. Sprinkle arrowroot power and sesame seeds (if desired) over the veggie then mix and remove from heat.

11. Serve with meatballs and hot sauce.

Nutritional Information: Calories: 486kcal; Total fat: 21.7g; Total carb: 53.1g; Protein: 16.9g

Fettuccine Pork-Belly Carbonara

Preparation time: 10 minutes

Cooking time: 15 minutes

Servings: 4

Ingredients:

1 lbs pork belly, fresh or cured (or bacon/pancetta)

1 pack Fettuccine, or any lectin free pasta of your choice

1/3 cup of grated Parmesan cheese/Parmigiano Reggiana

1 egg + 1 additional yolk, pasture raised

1 clove garlic

1 tsp black pepper or more

Salt (if meat isn't salted or cured)

Directions:

1. Get a pot of boiling water ready for the pasta. Note that the water should be ready before the pork is cooked. Fettuccine are ready in 90 minutes and don't look good when overcooked, so you need to be fast and precise.

2. Cook the pork belly cubes in a large sautéing or frying pan, big enough to contain the pasta. Add crushed garlic then mix regularly and cook at medium-low heat.

3. On the other hand, prepare the sauce base. Whisk the egg and extra yolk then add lots of pepper and grated cheese. Season with salt if the pork is salted or not cured. Whisk properly and set aside.

4. Immediately the pork belly is done, it should be crispy and most of its fat melted. Remove extra fat (store in a jar for other dishes), retaining enough to cover the pan and have a base for the sauce.

5. Take out the garlic clove then cook the pancetta or guaciale in olive oil, but with the pork belly isn't necessary.

6. Return the pork to the stove then set heat to the low. Add the pasta to the boiling water then leave for 90 seconds, not more.

7. After 90 seconds, add the pasta to the pork belly pan then add few tbsp of pasta water with it. Turn off the heat then place the pan to a non heated surface.

8. Mix egg and cheese mixture together then add it to the pasta and mix properly. Add few tbsp of pasta water if requited.

9. Serve at once.

Nutritional Information: Calories: 418kcal; Total fat: 21.7g, Total Carb: 36.2g; Protein: 19.4g

Creamy No-Lectin Shepherd's Pie

Preparation time: 30 minutes

Cooking time: 35 minutes

Servings: 4

Ingredients:

1 lbs grass fed ground lamb

½ cup goat's milk

½ cup of beef broth

2 sweet potatoes, diced

1 tablespoon olive oil

2 tablespoons chopped Italian parsley

1 yellow onion, diced

7 oz. cauliflower florets

1 big carrot, diced

3 garlic cloves with skins on

1 big celery stalk, chopped

3 sprigs thyme, remove the tem

6 tablespoons pastured butter

Pepper

Salt to taste

Directions:

1. Preheat oven to 375°F.

2. Dice the onions, carrot and sweet potatoes.

3. Heat up olive oil in a cast iron pot over medium-high heat. Add the carrots and sweet potatoes then cook for 10minutes.

4. Once the oven is preheated, set the cauliflower florets on a baking sheet, followed with the garlic, skin on.

5. Sprinkle olive oil, pepper and salt on top then bake in the oven 10 to 15 minutes until the cauliflower is al dente.

6. While the cauliflower is baking, dice the Italian parsley and celery.

7. Pour the chopped celery and onions into the pot then stir the veggies together.

8. Add the lamb then stir, breaking up the ground meat into small pieces. Keep cooking until the meat is browned.

9. Remove the baked cauliflower from the oven then set aside to cool. The oven should be kept on.

10. Pour the broth into the meat mixture. Add the herbs, reserving a few fresh thyme leaves for garnishing. Lower heat to a simmer, taste then season with pepper and salt.

11. Immediately the garlic and cauliflower has slightly cooled, take off garlic skins then throw them away.

12. Transfer cauliflower and garlic to the blender; add the melted butter and goat milk. Blend for few minutes until smooth.

13. Stir the veggies and meat together until it thickened. Its fine if there are some liquid in the pot.

14. Pour the meat mixture equally into 4 ramekins. Top each with cauliflower mixture then set each ramekin on a cookie sheet then bake for 30 to 35 minutes.

15. When the pies are done, allow them cool for 5 to 10 minutes.

16. Garnish with fresh thyme leaves then serve.

Nutritional Information: Calories: 624kcal; Total fat: 44g; Total carb: 25.5g; Protein: 32.3g

Slow Cooked Lemony Pork

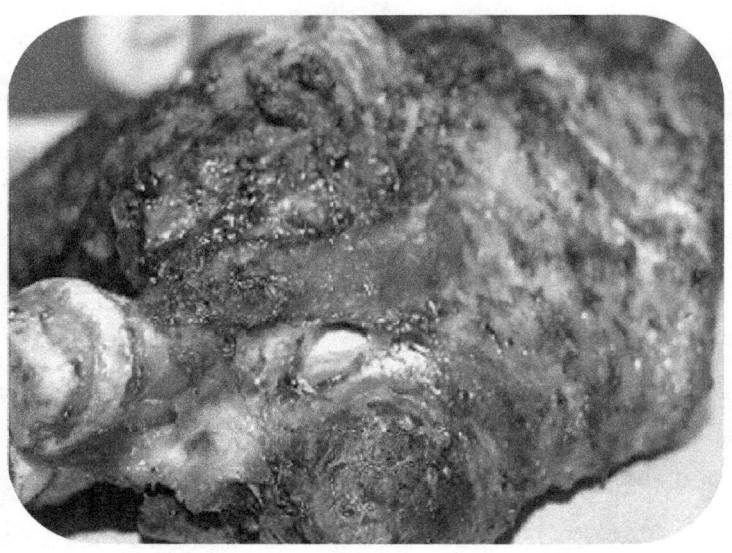

Preparation time: 30 minutes

Cooking time: 4 hours

Servings: 6

Ingredients:

1 rack pork ribs, pastured

5 cloves garlic, skins on

1 big sweet potato

2 tablespoon olive oil

4 cups chicken broth

Juice of 2 oranges

1 lime, juice

6 cloves garlic, finely chopped

1 lemon, juice

6 radishes, diced

1 yellow onion, sliced into rings crosswise

6 sprigs cilantro, chopped finely

1 teaspoon cumin

32 oz. cauliflower rice

1 teaspoon oregano

10 green olives, ground

1 avocado, diced

Pepper

Salt to taste

2 whole limes, quartered

Directions:

1. Pour olive oil into skillet then heat over medium-high heat.

2. Cut pork into two ribs or individual ribs then season each side with pepper and salt.

3. Add the pork ribs to the heated oil then brown each side for 2 to 3 minutes.

4. Chop the sweet potato into small cubes, dice the onions into thin rings then chop the garlic cloves.

5. Transfer the browned ribs to the slow cooker, followed with garlic and onions.

6. Squeeze out juices from lemon, oranges and lime into the slow cooker. Add the chicken stock then add 1 heaped spoon of spices.

7. Set the slow cooker to 8 hours on low or 4 hours on high.

8. Once its half hour before mealtime, heat up the oven to 375°F.

9. Heat up a cast iron pan with olive oil over medium-high heat.

10. Pour the cauliflower rice into the cast iron pan then stir for about 7 minutes until a just cooked.

11. Crush the green olives, this will release flavor. Add the olives and garlic with its skin removed to the cauliflower rice.

12. Transfer the cauliflower rice, with garlic and olives for 30 minutes.

13. Chop the avocado and radish then mince the fresh cilantro. Slice lime into quarter wedges.

14. Scoop the cauliflower into each serving bowls once it is baked. Pull out a veggie and ribs with tongs. Scoop out cooked juice over rice and pork.

15. Top with radish, cilantro and avocado then season with pepper and salt if desired. Garnish each serving bowl with lime wedges.

Nutritional Information: Calories: 837kcal; Total Fat: 48.7g; Total Carb: 36.4g; Protein: 66g

SEAFOOD RECIPES

Black Spiced Shrimp 'N' Alfredo Noodles

Enjoy an easy, delicious and of course a lectin-free dish of black spiced shrimp with creamy Alfredo noodle. The perfect meal for dinner time!

Preparation time: 10 minutes

Cooking time: 15 minutes

Servings: 2

Ingredients:

½ lb shrimp

1 tablespoon avocado oil

2 tablespoon of blackened spice

1 tablespoon butter

1/3-½ cup grated parmesan cheese

2 cups arugula (optional)

12 oz. (1 package) carrot noodles or any preferred noodles, cooked

2 minced garlic cloves

1 cup milk (cream for richer sauce)

Salt, to taste

Directions:

1. Rinse the shrimp, drain then coat in blackening spice.

2. Pour 1 tablespoon of avocado oil in a cast iron pan then heat over medium-high heat. Add the seasoned shrimp in the pan in a single layer.

3. Cook for 3 to 4 minutes, turning the shrimp gently with tongs and keep cooking for additional 3 to 4 minutes until well cooked and the spice is crusty then set aside.

4. Add 1 tablespoon of butter in a clean pan then melt over medium-high heat. Add the garlic then stir a bit until aromatic.

5. Pour in parmesan and a cup of cream or milk. Stir in slow motion until well heated and the cheese thicken the sauce.

6. Taste and season with salt if required. Make sure you taste before adding salt because parmesan can be salty.

7. Add the cooked noodles then stir until properly coated.

8. Serve with spiced shrimp and arugula on the side.

Nutritional Information: Calories: 469kcal; Total Fat: 24.9g; Total Carb: 23.1g; Protein: 38.9g

Green Curried Shrimp

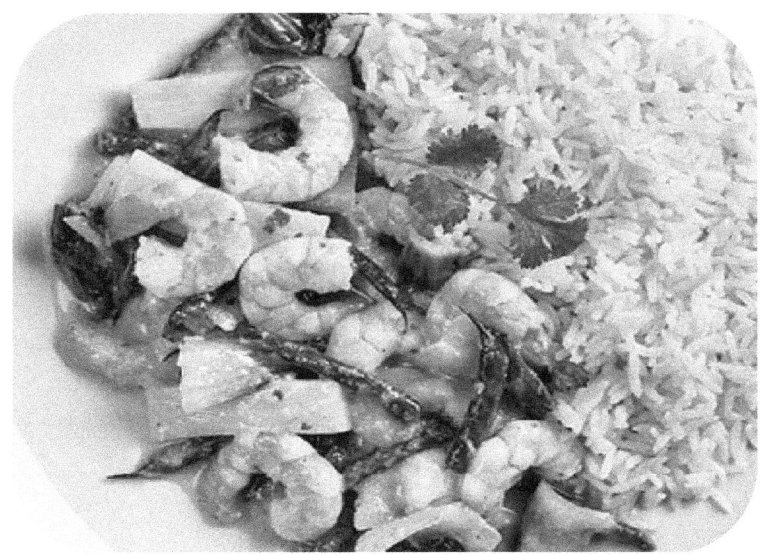

Whip up a flavorful green curry with shrimp. It's delicious, easy to make and yummy!

Preparation time: 10 minutes

Cooking time: 15 minutes

Servings: 2

Ingredients:

½ lb shrimp

2 tablespoons green curry paste

1½ tablespoon minced garlic (3 garlic cloves)

1 cup chopped white onion

½ tablespoon minced ginger

3 - 4 kaffir lime leaves

1 teaspoon avocado oil (or preferred oil)

For serving: 2 cups cauliflower rice

1 can of coconut milk

1 medium sweet potato, chopped then cooked

1 cup broccoli florets

Salt

For garnish: 1 tbsp scallions (optional)

Directions:

1. Boil the chopped sweet potato for 15 minutes or microwave for 5 minutes.

2. Pour oil into the pan then heat over medium high heat. Add the onion, ginger and garlic then cook for 3 minutes, stirring until translucent and aromatic.

3. Add the shrimp and stir. Season with a small pinch of salt and cook for about 30 seconds.

4. Add the cooked potatoes, coconut milk, broccoli and lime leaves/juice. Stir then simmer gently.

5. Add the green curry paste then stir until well mixed. Bring to a soft simmer then cook for about 6 to 7 minutes until the sauce is thickened.

6. Taste then add salt or additional green curry paste if you like. Garnish with scallions and serve over steamy cauliflower rice.

Nutritional Information: Calories: 582kcal; Total Fat: 32.9g; Total Carb: 43.8g; Protein: 33.5g

Broccoli Shrimp Stir Fry with Sesame Cauli Rice

Preparation time: 20 minutes

Cooking time: 30 minutes

Servings: 4

Ingredients:

10 oz broccoli, chopped into 2" pieces

1 lb wild-caught shrimp, peeled then deveined

½ head cauliflower rice

1 tbsp toasted sesame seeds + extra for serving

3 tbsp avocado oil

1 bunch scallions, chopped

1 tsp minced garlic

1 tbsp grated fresh ginger, 2" size

¼ cup rice vinegar

¼ cup veggie broth, unsalted

Directions:

1. Pour the cauli rice into a microwave-safe dish, cover and cook for 3 to 5 minutes. Now, stir in the sesame seeds.

2. While the cauli rice is cooking, in big skillet, heat up a tbsp of oil over med-high heat. Add the shrimp, cook, stirring from time to time for 2 to 4 minutes until opaque throughout. Once done, transfer to a plate; keep the skillet.

3. Pour the rest of the 2 tbsp of oil into the used skillet then add the broccoli, ginger and scallions, Cook for 8 to 10 minutes, stirring frequently, until the broccoli becomes soft.

4. Stir in the veggie broth and vinegar, tossing often for about 2 minutes until the sauce properly coats the veggies. Finally add the shrimp then toss for a minute.

5. Serve stir fry over the cauli rice then sprinkle sesame seeds on top.

Nutritional Information: Calories: 248kcal; Total Fat: 11.4g; Total Carb: 11.8g; Protein: 24.6g

Veggie Tuna Wrap

Preparation time: 15 minutes

Cooking time: 0 minute

Servings: 4

Ingredients:

2 (4.1 oz. cans) tuna, drained

1 celery, diced

1 big carrot, chopped

2 tbsp minced purple onion

¼ cup homemade mayonnaise

½ lemon, juice

¼ tsp black pepper

½ tsp sea salt

For the wraps: 4 romaine/iceberg lettuce leaves

Toppings (optional):

Avocado slices

Freshly cracked pepper

Minced purple onion

Red pepper flakes

Sliced black olives

Cilantro sprigs

Directions:

1. Combine tuna, mayonnaise, carrot, celery, lemon juice, onion, salt and black pepper in a large mixing bowl. Mix everything together with a wooden spoon.

2. Spread out the lettuce leaves then scoop large amount of tuna salad into the middle then top with preferred toppings.

3. You can add sliced olives, minced onion, cracked pepper, pepper flakes, cilantro sprigs and avocado slices. Fold the left leaf over the middle, followed with the right leaf over the left leaf. Enjoy.

4. Refrigerate left over tuna salad in a sealed container for up to 2 days.

Nutritional Information: Calories: 246kcal; Total Fat: 14.4g; Total Carb: 7.2g; Protein: 21.6g

Creamy Cilantro Salmon Burgers

Preparation time: 10 minutes

Cooking time: 1 hour + chilling time

Servings: 6 - 8 burgers

Ingredients:

1 lb wild caught salmon, ground or finely flaked

1/3 cup diced fresh cilantro

1 large egg, pastured

1/8 tsp red pepper flakes, crushed

1 tbsp organic coconut flour

¼ cup finely diced onion

1 garlic clove, pressed or minced

1 medium lime, juiced

1 tbsp mayonnaise (avocado oil)

½ tsp sea salt

Avocado oil spray

Directions:

1. Combine all the ingredients then and mix thoroughly.

2. Share mixture into 6 to 8 equal sizes then mold into patties.

3. Chill for an hour then grill over medium-high heat until well cooked, using avocado oil as required.

4. Serve and enjoy.

Nutritional Information: Calories: 105kcal; Total Fat: 5.8g; Total Carb: 2.1g; Protein: 12.1g

Avocado Veggie Shrimp Tostadas

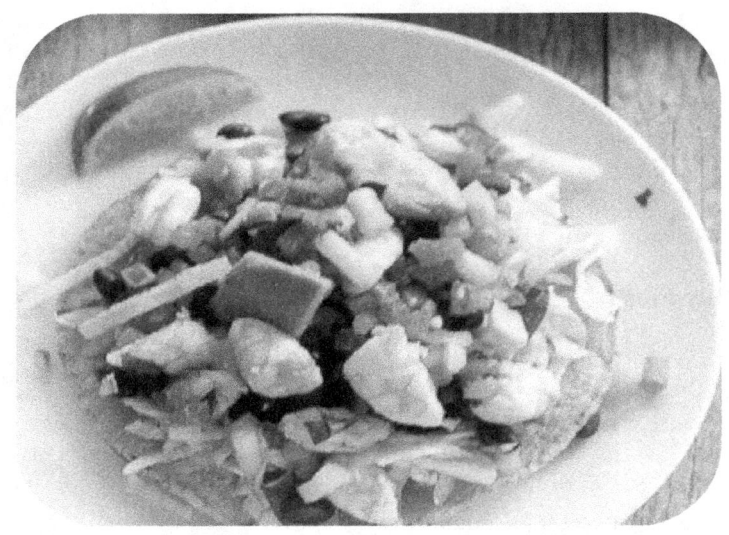

Preparation time: 15 minutes

Cooking time: 5 minutes

Servings: 2

Ingredients:

Avocado oil

4 almond flour tortillas

For the filling:

1 bunch of fresh cilantro, washed, dried and diced

½ small red cabbage, sliced finely

Thin slices of scallions or red onion, diced

1 avocado, sliced

Nutritional yeast

For serving: more lime

For the shrimps:

2 tablespoons extra virgin olive oil + more

2 cups cleaned wild caught shrimps

1 big garlic clove, crushed

Juice, 2 lemons

Spice mix: ¼ tsp of cayenne pepper (or more for spicy), ½ tsp of cumin and 1 tsp of dry oregano

Pepper

Salt

Directions:

1. Clean the pat the shrimps dry. Cut or leave them whole, this depend their size. Transfer them to a bowl.

2. Combine olive oil, lime juice, spice mix and smashed garlic in a small sauce bowl then mix.

3. Mix this mixture with the shrimp then refrigerate for 30 minutes or less.

4. Slice the cabbage finely then rub all over it. Chop the onion and cilantro then slice the avocado almost to the end then drizzle lime juice on it so it doesn't oxidize. Now, season with pepper and salt.

5. Preheat the oven to 350°F.

6. Lay 2 cooked tortillas on a large parchment lined sheet pan then brush both sides of the tortillas with a little avocado oil then put it in the oven for 5 minutes until crispy and hard, flipping them when its half time. Watch them closely so they don't burn. .

7. While the tortillas are baking, take out the shrimps then add them to a heated skillet with olive oil.

8. Stir and cook for some minutes, until pink and cooked in the middle.

9. Take out the tostadas, transfer to plates then add the fillings, starting wit the red cabbage, followed by the shrimps, cilantro, avocado and onion. Sprinkle nutritional yeast on top then add more lime if required.

Nutritional Information: Calories: 870kcal; Total Fat: 50.1g; Total Carb: 71.5g; Protein 41.6g

Italian-Style Seafood Nachos

Preparation time: 30 minutes

Cooking time: 20 minutes

Servings: 2 - 4

Ingredients:

For the seafood:

Extra virgin olive oil

1 lbs mixed or seafood medley

2 large garlic cloves, crushed

1 organic lemon, both zest and juice

Pepper

Salt

For the chips bed:

¼ - ½ cup grated Pecorino Romano

6 almond flour tortillas (or preferred lectin-free tortillas/tortilla chips)

For the toppings:

1 avocado

½ cup pitted olives

1 bunch cilantro

4 medium red radishes

1 small bunch scallions

1 lime

For the sauce:

Extra virgin olive oil

¼ cup goat yogurt

Spices: Sriracha, thyme, cumin, oregano, pepper and salt

Juices from seafood, cooked

Directions:

1. Preheat the oven to 350°F.

2. Get all the veggies ready by washing, drying and chop.

3. To make the tortillas chips; slice the tortillas into triangles then bake them at 350°F in a sheet pan for 5 minutes.

4. To prepare the seafood; whether fresh or frozen, wash and pat dry them with paper towels before you cook.

5. Heat up extra virgin olive oil in a sautéing or frying pan over low-medium heat. Add the crushed garlic then fry for about 3 minutes until aromatic. Add the seafood then cook for some minutes. Squeeze in lemon juice then sprinkle some lemon zest and then add pepper and salt. Don't overcook because they'll go to the oven for extra 10 minutes.

6. Take out the seafood, leaving the juices in the pan.

7. Prepare the sauce by mixing the juices from the pan with the remaining ingredients then add spices for your taste.

8. Line a sheet pan with parchment paper then set the tortilla chips on it. Top with Pecorino Romano and in between.

9. Add the veggies and seafood in layers. Reserve some scallions and fresh cilantro for garnishing. You can add radishes at the beginning or end.

10. Spoon some of the sauce on top then bake at 350°F for 10 minutes.

11. Take it out then sprinkle scallions and fresh cilantro on top. Serve with the remaining sauce and fresh lime.

Nutritional Information: Calories: 477kcal; Total Fat: 21.7g; Total Carb: 42.8g; Protein: 31.7g

Sardine Avocado Salad 'N' Greens

Preparation time: 15 minutes

Cooking time: 5 minutes

Serves: 2

Ingredients:

For the salad:

4.3 oz can of sardines, drained

1 avocado

1 teaspoon homemade mayo or store bought

Extra virgin olive oil

Lime juice

Green olives, pitted then sliced in half

Fresh cilantro

Salt to taste

Pepper

For the wraps:

Water, boiled

Lemon

4 big collard greens leaves

For the filling:

Fresh or fermented carrots

Broccoli, steamed

Pickled red onion

Directions:

1. Blanch the collard greens for 5 minutes in hot water with lemon. Take them out then pat dry.

2. Scrap the hard section of the stem with a good knife, ensuring the leaves aren't cut then put two leaves together.

3. Combine all the salad ingredients together then crush the sardines and avocado with a fork. Taste then season if required.

4. Top the two leaves with half of the salad. Add fermented carrots, broccoli and pickled onion.

5. Wrap the leaves around the filling, starting with the side then roll over the filling, just like a burrito. Continue with the other half. Once done, slice in half then serve.

Nutritional Information: Calories: 496kcal; Total Fat: 37.2g; Total Carb: 32.1g; Protein: 27.3g

Saucy Roasted Broccoli Tuna

Preparation time: 20 minutes

Cooking time: 30 minutes

Servings: 4

Ingredients:

2 (5 oz) cans tuna, finely chopped

9 oz Fettucine or preferred noodle

For the roasted broccoli:

1 tbsp avocado oil

1½ - 2 lbs broccoli florets

Pepper

Salt

For the sauce:

¾ cup minced onion

13.5 oz coconut milk or unsweetened almond

2 tbsp butter, grass fed (or avocado/coconut oil, ghee)

1 tbsp minced garlic

10.5 oz chicken/veggie broth

3 tbsp cassava flour

Freshly ground pepper

1 tsp salt

Directions:

1. To prepare the roasted broccoli; preheat the oven to 400°F.

2. Chop the broccoli into medium-sized florets then spray or toss with 1 tbsp of avocado oil. Season lightly with pepper and salt.

3. Transfer to a baking sheet lined with parchment paper, it should be large enough to occupy a single layer then roast in the oven for 20 minutes.

4. On a burner, set water for the pasta and bring to boil.

5. Chop the tuna or process it in a food processor, then set aside.

6. To make the sauce; Melt butter in a big saucepan or 12" skillet over medium heat.

7. Add the onion and cook for about 5 minutes, stirring at intervals until soft. Add the garlic then cook for additional 30 to 60 seconds until aromatic.

8. Add the cassava flour then reduce heat to medium low. Cook for a minute, stirring often until the flour turns golden brown.

9. Pour in the broth and coconut milk then Turn up heat back to medium high, stir until bubbling.

10. Reduce heat if required to maintain gentle boil for 2 to 3 minutes until sauce looks thickened. Turn the heat off

11. Add pepper, salt and tuna then mix to incorporate, cover to keep warm

12. Boil the pasta according to directions then drain.

13. Add pasta and roasted broccoli to the sauce then toss. Sprinkle nutritional yeast or parmigiano reggiano on top and serve.

Nutritional Information: Calories: 739kcal; Total Fat: 35.5g; Total Carb: 74g; Protein: 37.2g

Lectin-Free Decadent Mussels

Preparation time: 10 minutes

Cooking time: 10 minutes

Servings: 4

Ingredients:

1½ lbs mussels, de-beard then scrubbed lightly with water

2 tbsp butter, pastured

½ cup dry white wine

2 whole garlic cloves minced

2 whole shallots minced

½ cup Italian parsley, chop the leaves finely

Salt flakes to taste

Directions:

1. Scrub the mussels clean then set aside.

2. Melt butter in a Dutch oven or a big pot on the stovetop at medium-high.

3. Chop the garlic and shallots finely then add it to the pot. Stir with a wooden spoon.

4. Add the mussels once the mixture appears golden. Pour in the white wine then stir again.

5. Cover the pot with a lid then cook. Take off the lid after 3 to 5 minutes, the mussels should open up.

6. Remove the mussels from heat if majority have opened.

7. Transfer the mussels to a bowl with a spoon or tong. Scoop or ladle the garlic and shallot mixture all over the mussels, as much as you want, ensuring to get the tasty tidbits of garlic and shallot at the base then spread evenly over the mussels.

8. Chop some Italian parsley then sprinkle on top then add salt flakes.

Nutritional Information: Calories: 222kcal; Total Fat: 9.9g; Total Carb: 8.6g; Protein: 21.1g

Artichoke Kalamata Wild Cod

Preparation time: 20 minutes

Cooking time: 10 minutes

Servings: 2

Ingredients:

2 fillets cod, wild Alaskan

3 whole small artichoke heads, marinated

5 Kalamata olives

1 garlic clove

2 sprigs mint

1 tablespoon of Ghee

1½ tablespoon feta cheese (optional)

Pepper

Salt to taste

Directions:

1. Mince the garlic, olives and artichokes.

2. Melt ghee in a sauté pan for 1 to 2 minutes over medium-high heat.

3. Lay the fillets in the pan then add pepper. Don't add salt because the ingredients contain salt.

4. Cook the each side of the fillets for 2 minutes.

5. Chop the mint then set aside for garnish.

6. After 2 minutes flip over then continue cooking until golden brown and crispy.

7. Add the minced artichokes, garlic and olives, and cook for extra 2 minutes. If the fillets are very thick, cover the pan with a lid and cook throughout.

8. Once done, remove the pan from heat then transfer the fillets to a plate. Sprinkle cooked veggie accoutrement on top then garnish with feta cheese and mint. Season if needed.

Nutritional Information: Calories: 314kcal; Total Fat: 16.2g; Total Carb: 19.8g; Protein: 26.7g

SOUPS AND STEWS

Broccoli Beet Cleansing Soup

Preparation time: 15 mins

Cooking time: 1 hour

Servings: 2 - 4

Ingredients:

1 cup organic veggie broth

2 cups natural broccoli

3 cups filtered water

2 organic beets, chopped

10 organic garlic cloves, freshly smashed

2 carrots, sliced

1 organic red onion (diced)

½ tsp ground turmeric

1 tsp Himalayan pink salt

½ freshly squeezed lemon juice

2 organic bay leaves

½ tsp ground black pepper

½ tsp ground oregano

Directions:

1. Chop the carrots, broccoli, beets and onions into desired sizes.

2. Pour all the soup ingredients into a medium-size pot then bring to boil.

3. Reduce heat then simmer for an hour on low. Add seasonings to your taste.

Nutritional Information: Calories: 81kcal; Total Fat 0.4g; Total Carb 18g; Protein 3.3g

Creamy Veggie Mushroom Soup

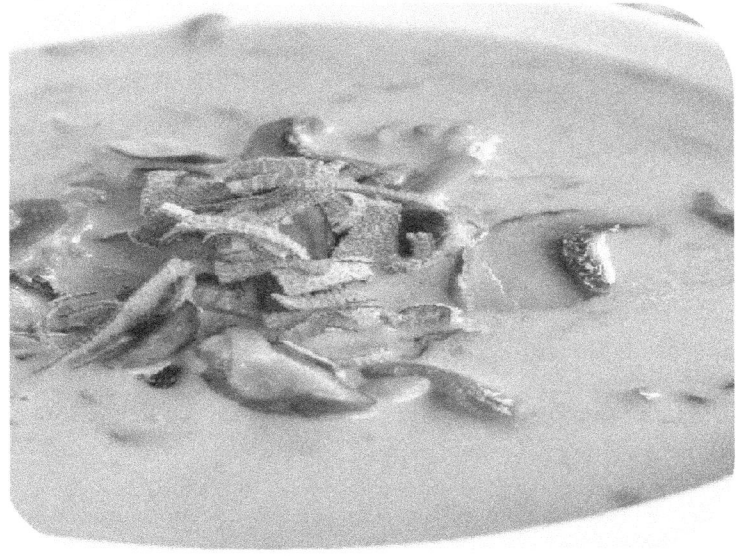

Preparation time: 10 minutes

Cooking time: 15 minutes

Servings: 2 - 4

Ingredients:

1 cup organic baby bella mushrooms, chopped

1 cup organic shitake mushrooms, chopped

1 cup veggie broth

½ cup red onions, organic, chopped

2 tsp pure avocado oil

13.5 oz. organic full-fat coconut milk

½ tsp Himalayan pink salt

1 freshly smashed garlic clove

½ tsp ground black pepper, organic

1 tbsp organic coconut aminos

½ tsp dried thyme

Directions:

1. Pour mushrooms, thyme, black pepper, garlic, pink salt, onions and avocado oil into a medium-size sauce pan.

2. Sauté for about 2 to 3 minutes on medium-high heat or until the mushrooms and onions are tender.

3. Pour in the veggie broth, coconut aminos and milk then stir. Taste and adjust seasonings to your desire.

4. Lower heat to medium-low then simmer for about 10 to 15 minutes, stirring often.

5. Decorate with extra mushroom slices, diced green onions and ground black pepper if desired. Serve.

6. Refrigerate leftover in an air-tight BPA-free container.

Nutritional Information: Calories 183kcal; Total Fat 16.7g; Total Carb: 8.3g; Protein: 2.7g

Chilled Mint-Berry Soup

Preparation time: 5 minutes

Cooking time: 5 minutes

Servings: 1 – 2

Ingredients:

For the soup:

8 organic fresh mint leaves

1 cup frozen organic berries: Blackberries, raspberries, blueberries

1 tsp freshly squeezed organic lemon juice

½ cup purified water

For the sweetener:

¼ cup of coconut sugar or Xylitol, non-GMO

¼ cup filtered water

Directions:

1. To prepare the sweetener: combine coconut sugar and water in a small saucepan and cook on low-medium heat, stirring for about 1 to 2 minutes until the sugar dissolves. Let it cool before adding to the soup.

2. To prepare the soup: Combine all the soup ingredients and sweetener in a blender, then process until well mixed.

3. Strain the soup through a strainer to separate seeds from the fruit. (reserve this to add to a smoothie later!)

4. Refrigerate in an air-tight BPA-free container. Enjoy!

Nutritional Information: Calories 110kcal; Total Fat 0.4g; Total Carb: 25.6g; Protein: 2.3g

Spiced Cauli-Rice Pumpkin Soup

Preparation time: 5 minutes

Cooking time: 10 minutes

Servings: 4 cups

Ingredients:

2 tsp organic pumpkin spice

13.5 oz. organic full-fat coconut milk

1 organic clove garlic, freshly smashed

4 cups of organic cauliflower rice

½ cup chopped organic red onion

2 tbsp extra-virgin olive oil

½ - 1 tsp Himalayan pink salt

1 tsp organic dried rosemary

½ tsp ground black pepper

Directions:

1. Combine olive, garlic, onions, rosemary, pepper and salt in a skillet then sauté for 2 to 3 minutes on medium heat until the onions are tender.

2. Add the cauli rice, pumpkin spice and all the coconut milk then stir until well mixed. Taste then adjust seasonings to your taste.

3. Simmer on low-medium heat if using frozen cauli rice, until the rice is thawed and soft.

4. Simmer on low-medium heat, if using raw cauliflower rice until soft.

5. Garnish with additional black pepper and dried rosemary if desired.

6. Serve warm. Enjoy!

Nutritional Information: Calories 324kcal; Total Fat 29.9g; Total Carb: 12.8g; Protein: 4.5g

Lectin-Free Vanilla Caramel Sauce

Preparation time: 5 minutes

Cooking time: 5 minutes

Servings: ½ cup

Ingredients:

½ cup almond butter, organic

½ tsp vanilla bean powder, organic

½ cup coconut oil, organic

1/8 tsp Himalayan pink salt

½ cup organic date nectar (or maple syrup)

Directions:

1. In a small bowl, combine all the ingredients then whisk everything together with a whisk until smooth, creamy and the oil is well combined.

2. Refrigerate in a BPA-free air-tight container or store in the pantry.

Note: If you refrigerate, it will turn thick and solidify due to the coconut oil. To thaw, run the container under warm water then stir again.

Nutritional Information: Calories 210kcal; Total Fat 18.6g; Total Carb: 7.9g; Protein: 3.5g

Creamy Veggie Asparagus Soup

Preparation time: 5 minutes

Cooking time: 5 minutes

Servings: 4 cups

Ingredients:

For the veggies:

12 stalks organic asparagus

3 freshly smashed organic garlic cloves

1 cup chopped organic onion

½ - 1 tsp Himalayan pink salt

2 tsp organic extra-virgin olive oil

½ - 1 tsp organic ground pepper

Other Ingredients:

13.5 oz. organic full-fat coconut milk

1 cup organic vegetable broth

Directions:

1. Prepare the sautéed veggies: chop the onion and slice the asparagus.

2. In a skillet, combine olive oil, asparagus, garlic, onions, black pepper and Himalayan pink salt the sauté on medium-high heat until the asparagus and onions becomes tender. Taste and adjust seasonings to taste.

3. Prepare the soup; pour all the coconut milk and veggie broth a blender, add the sautéed veggie then blend on "high" until smooth and creamy.

4. Warm soup on the stove top. Enjoy!

Nutritional Information: Calories: 420kcal; Total Fat: 39.5g; Total Carb: 9.4g; Protein: 4.9g

Lectin-Free Chicken Turmeric Soup

Preparation time: 10 minutes

Cooking time: 20 minutes

Servings: 3 - 4

Ingredients:

2½ teaspoon powdered turmeric

1/8 teaspoon powdered cayenne

1½ teaspoon powdered cumin

3 small chicken thighs, boneless

1 small onion, chopped

2 tablespoon coconut oil, butter or ghee, divided

4 cups diced veggies (broccoli, cauliflower and carrots)

1 cup of water

4 cups veggie/bone broth

1 bay leaf

½ cup full fat coconut milk (or preferred milk)

1 teaspoon grated fresh ginger

2 cups of chard, stem removed and sliced into thin rings

For garnishing: Lemon wedges, fresh cilantro and red pepper flakes

Directions:

1. In a small bowl, combine turmeric, cayenne and cumin then set aside.

2. Dice the chicken thighs with kitchen shears into small chunk sizes then set aside.

3. In a medium-sized soup pot, melt 1 tablespoon of preferred fat. Add onions then cook for about 3 minutes until translucent.

4. Add 4 cups of veggies and half of the turmeric mixture then cook for additional 3 to 4 minutes.

5. Add the broth, ginger, bay leaf and water then bring to boil. Reduce heat then simmer for 8 to 10 minutes until the veggies are fork tender. Turn the heat off then stir in the greens and coconut milk, let the green wilt.

6. While the veggies are cooking, melt the rest of the 1 tbsp of fat in a big skillet. Add chicken chunks then cook for about 5 minutes until its outside is no longer pink.

7. Add the rest of the turmeric mixture then cook for about 5 minutes until the chicken is well cooked in the inside.

8. Once veggies are cooked, scoop soup into bowls then top with cooked chicken and decorate with a squeeze of lemon, red pepper flakes and fresh cilantro.

Nutritional Information: Calories: 326kcal; Total Fat: 22.9g; Total Carb: 14.1g; Protein: 20.4g

Buttery Broccoli Cheddar Soup

Whip up a tasty lectin free buttery cheddar soup packed with broccoli and nutritional yeast. Enjoy.

Preparation time: 20 minutes

Cooking time: 20 minutes

Servings: 2

Ingredients:

1 large broccoli head, slice into florets

3 tbsp buttery coconut/olive oil

½ cup nutritional yeast

3 cups veggie broth

¼ cup arrowroot starch

¾ cup full-fat coconut milk

1 teaspoon Dijon mustard

¾ teaspoon salt

Directions:

1. Heat up a medium or large soup pot over medium heat.

2. Once heated, melt then add the arrowroot starch, whisk consistently for 3 to 4 minutes.

3. Now, whisk in the veggie broth slowly; add 1/3 cup of the broth in intervals, while whisking consistently before adding the next cup. This will prevent clumps from appearing.

4. Once half of the broth has been added, pour in the coconut milk, nutritional yeast, Dijon mustard, salt, and the remaining broth then bring to boil, stirring frequently.

5. Lower heat to medium-low then toss in the broccoli. Stir to coat the broccoli in broth then cover with a lid. Cook for about 10 minutes until soft to your liking.

6. Serve soup alone or with garlic muffins.

7. Refrigerate leftovers for up to 4 days. When ready to eat, reheat in a medium sauce pot over medium heat until it becomes bubbly.

Note: Par adventure, the broth ended up being clumpy, transfer the broth without broccoli to a blender then process for 30 seconds on high setting until smooth. Transfer the soup to the pot then add broccoli and continue with the cooking process.

Nutritional Information: Calories: 466kcal; Total Fat: 27.2g; Total Carb: 40.8g; Protein: 18g

Smoky Bean Miso-Mustard Greens Soup

Preparation time: 8 hours + soaking time

Cooking time: 1½ hours

Servings: 4 - 6

Ingredients:

4 cups mushroom broth

½ teaspoon of liquid smoke

1 lb mustard greens

1 tablespoon red miso paste

½ lb dry navy beans

4 large garlic cloves, crushed

½ yellow onion, chopped large

1 teaspoon paprika

1 tablespoon olive oil

2 cups water

Salt (a pinch)

Directions:

1. Soak navy beans in 2" of lukewarm water in a medium-sized bowl for 8 hours, covered with a plastic wrap or tea towel, changing the water halfway through. Drain then rinse the beans and set aside.

2. Clean the mustard greens thoroughly then take off most of their wooden stem. Slice the leaves in half then dice across horizontally to make big bands. Set aside.

3. Heat up a 6 qt pot or set an electric pressure-cooker to its sauté setting. Once it heated, add olive oil, onions, and a pinch of salt, cook for about 5 minutes until the edges are browned.

4. Add mustard greens, beans and the remaining ingredients to the pressure-cooker then stir for a minute thoroughly until combined.

5. Cover with the cooker's lid and cook on high 40 minutes. After 40 minutes, let the pressure release on its own for 30 to 45 minutes.

6. Once the pressure has been released, serve.

7. Refrigerate leftovers in an airtight container for up to 6 days. Once ready to eat, reheat in a medium pot over medium-low heat until heated.

8. Top with Sriracha hot sauce and nutritional yeast.

Note: Sauté the onions over medium-high heat, if you are using a manual pressure cooker. If using an electric pressure cooker, cook the onions over medium-high heat till it turns brown before transferring to the cooker.

If you don't have a pressure cooker, use two 15 oz canned navy beans in place of dried beans. Cook soup over medium-low heat at a gentle simmer for 45 minutes until the greens are very soft.

Nutritional Information: Calories 183kcal; Total Fat 3.1g; Total Carb: 29.4g; Protein: 12.1g

Shiitakei Spicey Sour Soup

Preparation time: 20 minutes

Cooking time: 1 hour

Servings: 3

Ingredients:

6 oz shiitake mushrooms, cut about ¼" thick

7 cups of water

1 (1") ginger, julienned

¾ oz black fungus, dried

2 teaspoons toasted sesame oil

2 large cloves garlic, sliced thinly

¾ teaspoon ground white pepper

2 bouillon cubes

¼ cup rice vinegar

1 tablespoon tamari

2 tablespoons tapioca starch plus 3 tablespoons of water

1 teaspoon chili paste or more

For topping: scallions, sliced thinly

Directions:

1. Soak black fungus in hot water in a medium-sized mixing bowl then let it sit for 20 to 30 minutes. Meanwhile prepare other ingredients.

2. Shake tapioca and 3 tablespoons of water vigorously in a small air-tight container then set aside.

3. Heat up a big soup pot over high heat then add sesame oil, mushrooms and a pinch of salt. Cook both sides until browned, stirring occasionally.

4. Add the soaked fungus and other ingredients except the scallions and starch mixture then bring to boil.

5. Reduce heat to medium-low then simmer for 30 minutes. Add the starch mixture then bring to boil over high heat.

6. Once it boils, turn off heat. Serve with fresh scallions

7. Refrigerate leftovers in an air-tight container for up to 3 days. Once read to eat, re-heat in a pot over medium heat until heated.

Nutritional Information: Calories: 90kcal; Total Fat 3.6g; Total Carb: 11.9g; Protein: 2.5g

Beef Chili

Preparation time: 15 minutes

Cooking time: 6 hours

Servings: 8

Ingredients:

2 lbs grass-fed ground beef

1 tbsp avocado oil divided

4 garlic cloves, minced

3 ribs celery, chopped finely

1 medium onion, chopped finely

2 tbsp powdered chili

¼ tsp ground cinnamon

2 tsp ground cumin

3 oz. pine nuts

1 pinch ground cloves

2 cups grass-fed beef broth

1 tbsp adobo sauce from preserved chipotles

2 tsp red wine vinegar

15 oz. canned sweet potato puree

2 tsp coconut aminos

For serving: Full fat sour cream, organic

For garnish: lime wedges, scallion slices

Directions:

1. In a big non-stick skillet, heat up 1 tsp of oil over high heat. Add 1 lb of ground beef and ½ tsp of salt then brown, breaking the meat with a spatula for 3 to 4 minutes. Transfer to the pot then repeat with the rest of the beef.

2. Reduce the heat to medium then heat the rest of the tsp of oil. Add the onion, garlic, and celery then cook for 5 minutes until tender.

3. Add the powdered chili, cloves, cinnamon and cumin then stir, cooking for a minute. Add broth, scrape the base of the pan then transfer to the slow cooker pot.

4. Add the sweet potato puree, pine nuts, coconut aminos, wine vinegar, adobo sauce, pepper and 2 tsp of salt. Cover then slow cook for 6 hours on medium setting. make sure the knob is turned to vent the steam.

5. Serve with lime wedges, scallions and sour cream, if desired.

Nutritional Information: Calories: 231kcal; Total Fat: 14g; Total Carb: 16.7g; Protein: 11.3g

Cauli Shrimpy Soup

Preparation time: 25 minutes

Cooking time: 35 minutes

Servings: 4

Ingredients:

1 cup frozen mini shrimps, wild-caught, cooked

7 medium raw whole shrimps, wild-caught, with skin and heads

13 oz cauliflower rice

1 peeled garlic clove

3 tbsp red palm oil

1 leek, white part

1 pinch of aniseeds

2 (13.5 oz.) cans full fat coconut milk, non BPA

1 tbsp Hungarian paprika

1 lime

1 fresh bunch cilantro, diced

Pepper

Salt

Directions:

1. Sauté each side of the whole shrimps in red palm oil for some minutes, you may cover the pot after turning them. Once completely pink, transfer to a plate.

2. In the same oil, add the diced leek then sauté for some minutes. Add the peeled and crushed garlic and aniseed then sauté for some minutes.

3. Add half of the cauliflower then sauté for some minutes. Add the paprika, pepper and salt.

4. Add 1 can of coconut milk, the whole shrimps including the skin and heads then bring to boil. Simmer for some minutes until the cauliflower is cooked.

5. Remove the shrimps then transfer the soup to a blender then blend until smooth. Transfer back to the pot.

6. Add the remaining cauliflower and the other can of coconut milk then simmer on low heat.

7. While its cooking, peel and devein the shrimps then slice into bite size chunks, keeping one or two unpeeled for garnishing.

8. Add the frozen, cooked mini shrimps to the soup then add the sliced shrimps, diced cilantro and juice from ½ lime or extra to taste.

9. Taste and add pepper and salt or more if required. Serve warm with lime.

Nutritional Information: Calories: 985kcal; Total Fat: 81.7g; Total Carb: 25.7g; Protein: 42.1g

Veggie Beef Stew

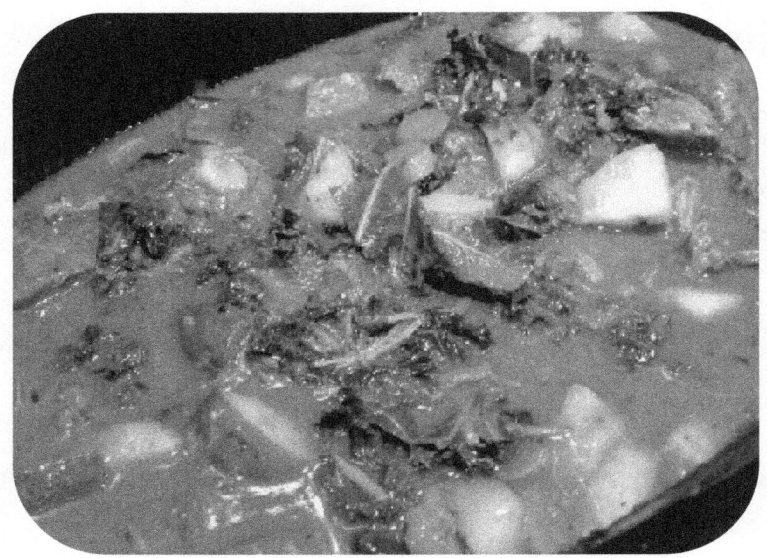

Preparation time: 1 hour

Cooking time: 2 hours

Servings: 6

Ingredients:

1½ lbs beef, grass-fed

2 big parsnips (or more if small), peeled then diced into small chunks

¼ cup extra virgin olive oil, or more if required

2 cups beef stock

3 medium sunchokes, peeled then chopped into medium chunks

1 big turnip, peeled then chop roughly into big chunks

2 medium sweet onions, chopped roughly

6 peeled cloves garlic, minced

1 - 2 cups of water

3 small spring onions, diced into ½" pieces

½ cup of red wine

2 bay leaves

1 bunch of fresh parsley, diced

½ tsp of all spice

1 tsp of dry thyme

¼ tsp of nutmeg

1 tbsp of Hungarian paprika

1 tbsp of powdered arrowroot

Pepper

Salt

Directions:

1. Heat up oil in the pan over medium heat.

2. Slice the beef in cubes then sprinkle with salt. Pat dry with a paper towel then brown them in batches.

3. Once it's browned, transfer them back to the pot then add the garlic. Sauté for about 40 seconds until aromatic, then add the beef stock, water and red wine. Bring to a boil then add thyme, nutmeg and all spice, cover then simmer for 1 hour 15 minutes on the lowest heat.

4. Once the simmering time is almost done, start preparing the veggies. Pour olive oil in the pan then sauté parsnips and two onions for about 10 minutes.

5. Add the paprika then mix properly so the paprika doesn't burn, add a couple of tbsp of water then add the turnips and sunchockes. Mix properly then sauté for some minutes.

6. Add the veggies to the pot containing meat then simmer uncovered for about 45 minutes. Now add pepper and salt to taste.

7. Once done, take off some of the fat on top, if you want then add the thickener (powdered arrowroot + cold water then mixed with 1 tbsp of ho stew liquid) then simmer for another 5 minutes.

8. Add the spring onion and fresh parsley.

9. Serve soup with steamed veggies or raw cabbage salad.

Nutritional Information: Calories: 387kcal; Total Fat: 20.9g; Total Carb: 22g; Protein: 25.9g

Creamy Root Veggie Soup

Preparation time: 20 minutes

Cooking time: 35 minutes

Servings: 4

Ingredients:

½ medium sweet potato, chopped

1 small rutabaga, chopped

2 big celery sticks, diced

1 medium red onion, diced

¼ cup extra virgin olive oil

½ big celeriac, chopped

1 big parsnip, diced

Fresh thumb-size ginger, diced

1 fennel stick, diced

3 - 4 stems of fresh thyme

1 big peeled garlic clove, crushed

Juice of ½ lemon

Fresh thumb-size turmeric, diced

1 bay leaf

Iodized sea salt

Pepper to taste

1 tsp of nutritional yeast

Hot water

Directions:

1. In a soup pot, heat olive oil over medium heat then add celery and onions then sauté for some minutes.

2. Add garlic and the remaining veggies then mix properly. Cover the pot then cook for about 5 minutes. Uncover the pot and re-mix, cover for additional 5 minutes. Repeat this process few more times. All the veggies should cook in the olive oil and steam.

3. After 15 minutes, add the bay leaf, thyme, pepper and salt then cover the veggies with hot water. Cover then simmer for another 15 minutes, or until the veggies are tender but not overcooked.

4. Transfer to a food processor then process until smooth. Transfer back to the soup pot then add more hot water if it's very thick.

5. Taste then season with nutritional yeast, pepper if required and more salt. Squeeze in fresh lemon juice to taste.

Nutritional Information: Calories: 219kcal; Total Fat: 13.8g; Total Carb: 24g; Protein: 3g

VEGETABLE RECIPES

Roasted Cauli Rice

Treat yourself to simple roasted cauliflower rice garnished with fried eggs and green onions. Tasty!

Preparation time: 5 minutes

Cooking time: 25 minutes

Servings: 2

Ingredients:

1 head cauliflower, riced

½ teaspoon powdered garlic

2 tablespoons avocado oil

½ teaspoon powdered onion

1 teaspoon paprika

¼ teaspoons turmeric, optional

Sesame seeds, optional

Pepper

Sea salt to taste

Fried eggs (or pan-fried tofu), if desired

Green onions, sliced

Sriracha

Directions:

1. Heat up oven to 425°F. Line 13 by 8" rimmed baking sheet with parchment paper.

2. Spread the riced cauliflower on the lined baking sheet then add oil and seasonings, pepper and salt included, stir to combine.

3. Bake for 12 minutes then stir. Return to oven then bake for another 10 to 13 minutes until golden and begins to turn crispy. Watch closely so it doesn't burn.

4. Serve with tofu or fried eggs, sesame seeds, green onion slices and a drizzle of sriracha.

Note: You may core the cauliflower, rinse then process in a blender until you get desired consistency.

Nutritional Information: Calories: 234kcal; Total Fat: 19.2g; Total Carb: 12.7g; Protein: 6g

Feta Olives Filled Wraps

You can't go wrong with these soft and flavorful wraps filled with hummus, olives, guacamole and feta.

Preparation time: 5 minutes

Cooking time: 25 minutes

Servings: 3 wraps

Ingredients:

½ cup almond flour

6 tablespoons arrowroot flour

1 tablespoon coconut flour

2 tablespoons nutritional yeast

¼ teaspoon powdered garlic

1 teaspoon za'atar, if desired

1 cup coconut milk

1½ teaspoon coconut oil, for cooking

¼ teaspoon sea salt

Directions:

1. Whisk all the ingredients except coconut milk and oil in a small mixing bowl.

2. Add the coconut milk then whisk to combine.

3. In a medium skillet, heat up ½ tsp of coconut oil over medium heat until it melt then swirl the oil around the pan.

4. Pour ½ cup of the mixture into the center of the pan then turn the pan so the batter can spread. Cook for 5 to 7 minutes until the first side begins to turn golden brown.

5. Flip then cook the other side for another 3 to 5 minutes until golden brown and starts to puff up. Take out from the pan then cool while you cook the other wraps.

Note: for quick and easy measuring, 6 tbsp is the same as ¼ cup plus 2 tbsp.

Nutritional Information: Calories: 327kcal; Total Fat: 24.6g; Total Carb: 24.4g; Protein: 6.8g

Sautéed Veggie Bowl

Preparation time: 5 minutes

Cooking time: 15 minutes

Servings: 2 - 4

Ingredients:

6 oz fresh baby spinach

10 oz mushrooms

1 tbsp. olive oil

1 tsp. coconut aminos

Pepper

Salt

1 - 2 garlic cloves

1 tsp. sherry vinegar

2 tsp. of nutritional yeast

Red pepper flakes or Aleppo pepper (optional)

Directions:

1. Wash the mushrooms then slice thinly and set aside. Chop the garlic finely or make use i\of a garlic press then set aside.

2. Heat up a big non-stick skillet over medium heat. Add olive oil then let i heat for a minute then add the mushroom slices. Toss with oil to coat then cook for a minute. Season pepper and salt to taste.

3. Cook the mushrooms for about 10 minutes, stirring constantly until a reasonable amount of liquid is released. You can increase heat to medium-high.

4. Add the fresh spinach then toss with the mushrooms until the spinach is a bit wilted then season again with pepper and salt.

5. Add the coconut aminos, nutritional yeast and sherry vinegar then stir to mix well. Once the sherry evaporates, create a space then add the garlic directly to the pan and cook for about 30 seconds until aromatic, stir to mix with the spinach and mushrooms.

6. Sprinkle pepper flakes or Aleppo pepper on top if desired. Serve.

Note: You can use baby bella or Portobella mushrooms. You can also use tamari in place of coconut aminos, but reduce the salt because tamari contains a lot more sodium.

Nutritional Information: Calories: 66kcal; Total Fat: 4g; Total Carb: 5.4g; Protein: 4.3g

Brussels Berry Salad 'N' Balsamic Vinaigrette

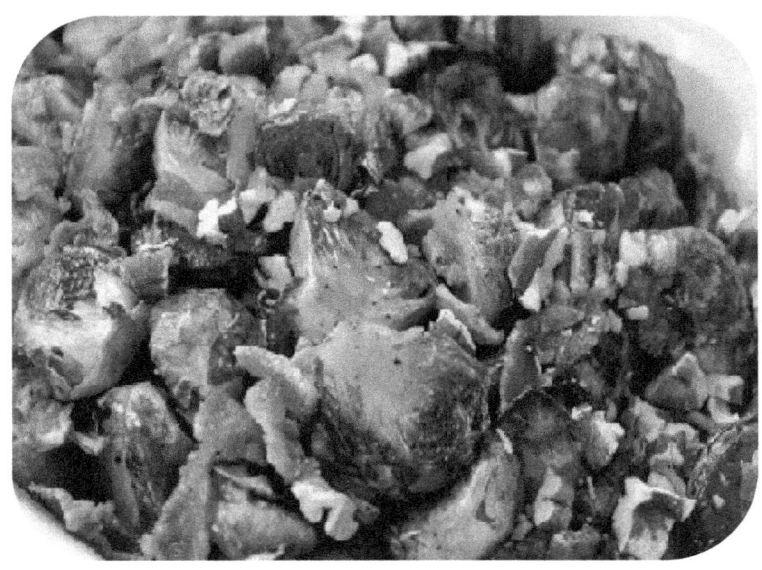

Whip up a quick salad and dressing in 5 minutes.

Preparation time: 5 minutes

Cooking time: 0 minute

Servings: 4

Ingredients:

10 oz. shaved Brussels sprouts

½ cup dried cranberries

½ cup raw walnuts, diced roughly

½ cup chopped green onions

Dressing:

1 tbsp + 1 tsp of maple syrup

3 tbsp fresh lemon juice

1 tbsp whole grain mustard

2 tbsp avocado oil

Ground black pepper, to taste

¾ tsp of sea salt

Directions:

1. Prepare the dressing; whisk all the ingredients together in a mixing bowl until emulsified or shake in a glass jar with a tight closed lid then set aside.

2. Add the shaved Brussels sprouts then toss with dressing.

3. Add the diced walnuts, onion slices and dried cranberries then toss to combine.

Note: Save time by buying already shaved Brussels with no sugar. Use desired sugar substitute.

Nutritional Information: Calories 237kcal; Total Fat: 17.3g; Total Carb: 20.5g; Protein: 5.1g

Roast-y Sweet Potatoes 'N' Arugula Salad

A combination roasted sweet potatoes with spicy arugula and creamy goat cheese. Yummy!

Preparation time: 10 minutes

Cooking time: 35 minutes

Servings: 2

Ingredients:

2 small peeled sweet potatoes, sliced into small chunks

2½ oz Arugula

2 tbsp avocado/olive oil

1 tbsp Balsamic vinaigrette

2 tsp Herbs de Provence

1 oz soft goat cheese

Pepper

Salt

Directions:

1. Heat up the oven to 400°F.

2. In a half sheet baking pan, toss the cubed sweet potatoes with avocado/olive oil, pepper, herbs de Provence and salt then bake for 20 minutes. Stir and cook for another 10 to 15 minutes until the potatoes are soft in the center. Set aside to cool.

3. Toss the arugula with balsamic vinaigrette then share onto plates then top with roasted potatoes and cheese.

4. Serve and enjoy!

Nutritional Information: Calories: 892kcal; Total Fat: 63.1g; Total Carb: 58.6g; Protein: 25.9g

Vinegar Broccoli Shallot Salad

Make a lectin free salad with just seven ingredients and can be easily doubled for a large serving size.

Preparation time: 5 minutes

Cooking time: 10 minutes

Servings: 2 - 3

Ingredients:

¼ cup olive oil

1 head broccoli, sliced into small florets

2 tbsp white wine vinegar

1 shallot, sliced into thin rounds

¼ cup pistachios, diced roughly

1½ tsp. dijon mustard

Pepper to taste

Salt

Directions:

1. Blanch the broccoli.

2. Fill a medium-sized pot with cold water then bring to a boil and then season with salt. Once it starts boiling, add the broccoli florets for a minute. Plunge them immediately into an ice water bath to end cooking process then set aside.

3. In a mason jar, combine oil, shallots, mustard, vinegar, pepper and salt then shake to combine.

4. Drain the broccoli properly then dry with a paper towel if required.

5. Toss the broccoli with dressing

6. When ready to serve, top with diced pistachios.

Nutritional Information: Calories: 220kcal; Total Fat: 19.5g; Total Carb: 10.8g; Protein: 4.3g

Lectin-Free Lime Cilantro Cauli-Rice
Preparation time: 5 minutes

Cooking time: 5 minutes

Servings: 1½ cups

Ingredients:

For the cauliflower rice:

1 tbsp pure avocado oil

2 cups organic cauliflower rice

½ tsp organic ground black pepper

2 tbsp organic lime juice

1 tsp Himalayan pink salt

Other Ingredient:

¼ cup chopped organic fresh cilantro

Directions:

1. In a skillet, combine all the cauliflower rice ingredients then sauté lightly for about 5 minutes or until you achieve the texture you like. Adjust seasonings to your desire.

2. Remove from heat then add the diced cilantro then stir until equally distributed

3. Scoop into serving dish then decorate with the remaining diced cilantro.

4. Enjoy!

Nutritional Information: Calories: 99kcal; Total Fat: 7g; Total Carb: 7.3g; Protein: 2.2g

Roast-y Artichoke Greens Salad 'N' Sesame Seed Dressing
Preparation time: 5 minutes

Cooking time: 30 minutes

Servings: 1 - 2

Ingredients:

For the artichokes:

1 tbsp pure avocado oil

14 oz. canned artichoke hearts, drained

For the salad:

2 - 4 cups organic mixed salad greens

For the dressing:

2 tbsp pure avocado oil

1 tbsp organic sesame seeds

2 tbsp organic apple cider vinegar

1 tbsp organic date nectar

1 organic shallot, chopped

1/8 tsp organic black ground pepper

1/8 tsp Himalayan pink salt

For the seasoning:

1/8 tsp organic ground powdered garlic

1/8 tsp Himalayan pink salt

1/8 tsp organic ground paprika

1/8 tsp organic ground black pepper

Directions:

1. Preheat the oven to 425°F.

2. Prepare the seasoning: combine all the seasonings in a small bowl then stir.

3. Adjust the seasonings to taste then set aside.

4. Prepare the artichokes: Drain the artichokes then chop off the tips then slice into quarter or half pieces.

5. Toss artichokes and avocado oil together in a medium-sized bowl until coated and well incorporated.

6. Sprinkle evenly with seasoning then toss gently to ensure all the pieces are well coated with seasoning.

7. Transfer the seasoned pieces to a parchment paper lined baking pan then roast for 25 to 30 minutes at 425°F. Toss them halfway through cooking time and ensure they don't over bake or burn.

8. Prepare the dressing; combine all the dressing ingredients in a small bowl then whisk together until well combined.

9. Season to taste then set aside.

10: To assemble; Scoop 1 to 2 handfuls of mixed salad greens to serving dish then top with roasted artichokes.

11. Add any other desired topping of your choice like hemp seeds, slivered almonds, red onions, sesame seeds etc.

12. Drizzle sesame seed dressing on top. Enjoy!

Nutritional Information: Calories: 827kcal; Total Fat: 24.3g; Total Carb: 160.8g; Protein: 12g

Cauli-Rice Mushroom Risotto

Preparation time: 10 minutes

Cooking time: 10 minutes

Servings: 2 cups

Ingredients:

2 tbsp organic extra-virgin olive oil

1½ cups chopped organic baby bella mushrooms

½ tsp organic ground sage

½ cup chopped organic red onion

1 tsp organic ground black pepper

2 organic garlic cloves, freshly smashed

1 tsp Himalayan pink salt

Other Ingredients:

4 cups organic cauliflower rice

13.5 oz. organic full-fat coconut milk

Directions:

1. Make an advanced preparation by refrigerating a can of full-fat coconut milk overnight.

2. Prepare the veggies by chopping the mushrooms and onions into small pieces.

3. In a skillet, combine all the ingredients except coconut milk and cauliflower rice then sauté on medium-high heat until the mushrooms and onions are soft.

4. Take out the canned coconut milk from the refrigerator then scoop out the coconut fat. Don't use coconut water, reserve to make a smoothie later. Note that the more liquid added the less thick the risotto will be.

5. Add the cauliflower rice and coconut fat to the skillet then stir until everything is incorporated.

6. Simmer on medium heat until the cauliflower is softened to rice texture.

7. Adjust seasonings to your taste. Enjoy!

Nutritional Information: Calories: 635kcal; Total Fat: 49.4g; Total Carb: 33.6g; Protein: 13.2g

Spicy Avocado 'N' Roasted Potato Salad and Lime Tahini Dressing

Preparation time: 10 minutes

Cooking time: 25 minutes

Servings: 1 - 2

Ingredients:

For the sweet potatoes:

1 tbsp pure avocado oil

2 cups organic sweet potato cubes

¼ - ½ tsp ground powdered garlic

1 tsp organic ground powdered chipotle

1 cup organic spring salad mix

¼ tsp Himalayan pink salt

For the topping:

½ - 1 organic avocado cubes

1 - 2 tbsp chopped organic red onions

For the dressing:

2 tbsp filtered water

¼ cup organic tahini

¼ tsp organic powdered ground garlic

3 tbsp organic lime juice

1 - 2 pinch of organic ground black pepper

¼ tsp Himalayan pink salt

Directions:

1. Preheat the oven to 350°F.

2. Prepare the potatoes; peel the sweet potatoes then chop into cubes.

3. Pour the potato cubes into a medium-sized bowl then toss with avocado oil until well coated.

4. Combine garlic powder, chipotle powder and pink salt in a small bowl, stir until well mixed.

5. Sprinkle seasoning mix over sweet potato cubes then toss until well coated. Adjust seasonings to your taste.

6. Transfer the seasoned sweet potato cubes to a parchment paper line baking pan then bake for about 25 minutes at 350°F until soft.

7. Meanwhile prepare the dressing; combine all dressing ingredients in a small bowl then whisk until everything is well combined. Adjust seasonings to your taste then set aside.

8. Prepare the toppings; chop the avocado and red onion then set aside.

9. To assemble; Divide spring salad mix, or desired greens amongst serving plates then sprinkle chopped avocado and red onions on top.

10. Once the potatoes are ready, place them on top of the salad then ladle dressing over the salad. Serve warm and enjoy!

Nutritional Information: Calories: 449kcal; Total Fat: 29.8g; Total Carb: 42.2g; Protein: 10.9g

Peach Berry Salad 'N' Ginger Tahini Dressing

Preparation time: 10 minutes

Cooking time: 0 minute

Servings: 4

Ingredients:

For the salad:

8 handfuls organic spring salad mix

2 cups organic peaches/ mango, peeled then chopped into cubes

2 cups organic blueberries

1 cup of organic pecans

For the dressing:

½ cup organic date nectar

½ cup organic tahini

8 - 10 tbsp purified water

½ tsp organic ground ginger

Directions:

1. Prepare the dressing; combine all the dressing ingredients in a small bowl then whisk until well mixed. Adjust sweetener to your taste then adjust water to achieve desired texture.

2. To assemble; scoop 2 handfuls of spring salad mix to each serving plate then sprinkle ¼ of the blueberries on top, followed with ¼ of the pecans and ¼ of the chopped peaches/mango.

3. Ladle the ginger tahini dressing on top, dividing equally between the salad portions. Enjoy!

Nutritional Information: Calories: 537kcal; Total Fat: 38.8g; Total Carb: 47.8g; Protein: 12.2g

SNACK AND DESSERT RECIPES

Tasty Cheese Nachos

Preparation time: 15 minutes

Cooking time: 10 minutes

Servings: 1½ cup

Ingredients:

¼ cup avocado oil

1 cup peeled sweet potato cubes

3 tbsp white vinegar

½ cup peeled, diced carrot

2 tbsp nutritional yeast

¼ cup coconut milk

1 tsp powdered garlic

2 tbsp hot sauce

½ tsp of sea salt

1 tsp. of powdered onion

Directions:

1. Boil carrots and sweet potatoes for 10 minutes until fork tender then drain, reserve liquid and set aside.

2. Pour all the rest of the ingredients except liquid from potatoes and carrots into a blender. Add the cooked carrots and sweet potatoes then

blend until extremely smooth. Add a little of the kept liquid thin out into desired texture, if required.

3. Warm up the cheese gently for 15 to 30 seconds in the microwave or on the stove, stirring in between. Serve with preferred nacho toppings or chips.

Note: You may substitute hot sauce for ¼ to ½ tsp of cayenne pepper, this depends on your desired spice taste. You can make your own chips with plantain, cassava flour or yucca chips.

Nutritional Information: Calories: 746kcal; Total Fat: 77.5g; Total Carb: 15.4g; Protein: 1.6g

Black Peppercorn Sesame Turmeric Crackers

Preparation time: 5 minutes

Cooking time: 20 minutes

Servings: 40 - 50 crackers

Ingredients:

For the cracker:

1 tbsp organic coconut oil

1¾ cup almond flour

1 tbsp ground flax seeds plus 3 tbsp purified water (1 flax egg)

¼ cup nutritional yeast

1 tsp ground turmeric, organic

½ tsp ground garlic, organic

½ cup sesame seeds, organic

½ tsp ground black pepper, organic

½ tsp Himalayan pink salt

For the toppings:

Black peppercorn, freshly ground

Coarse Himalayan pink salt, freshly ground

Directions:

1. Preheat the oven to 350°F.

2. Prepare the flax egg; mix ground flax seeds and water in a small bowl then whisk until well mixed then set aside.

3. Meanwhile, prepare the cracker mixture. Combine the rest of the cracker ingredients in a medium-sized bowl then stir until well mixed.

4. Whisk the flax egg again then mix it with the cracker mixture then stir everything together until well mixed. Note that the batter should be crumbly and a bit moist.

5. Transfer the cracker batter to parchment paper lined baking pan.

6. Gather the batter then mold into a ball shape, squeeze tightly and compact.

7. Cover the cracker balls with a piece of parchment paper then press down so the flattened cracker is in between the parchment papers.

8. Flatten the cracker with a rolling pin into a square shape about 7 by 11" size. Take off the parchment paper on top then slice the dough with a butter knife or pizza cutter into small squares.

9. Sprinkle ground black peppercorn, pink salt with a grinder on top.

10. Place the baking pan in the oven for about 20 to 25 minutes at 350°F, watching them closely so they don't burn.

11. Take out the pan from the oven then flip over the crackers then bake for another 5 minutes, watching them closely so they don't burn.

12. Store in a BPA-free air-tight container. Enjoy!

Nutritional Information: Calories: 105kcal; Total Fat: 8.2g; Total Carb: 7.1g; Protein: 4.6g

Turmeric Spiced Potato Fries

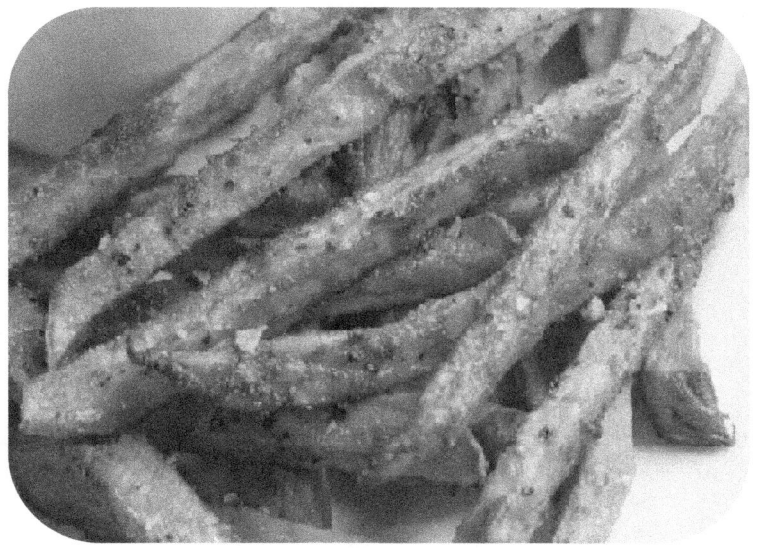

Preparation time: 5 minutes

Cooking time: 20 minutes

Servings: 50 - 60 fries

Ingredients:

1 tbsp pure avocado oil

1 large sweet potato, organic

For the seasoning:

½ tsp organic powdered turmeric

½ tsp organic ground black pepper

½ tsp organic cayenne pepper

2 tbsp nutritional yeast

½ tsp Himalayan pink salt

Directions:

1. Preheat the oven to 425°F.

2. Prepare the sweet potato; peel the sweet potato then slice off the ends then slice down the middle from top to bottom.

3. Slice the potato into French fries length. This should make about 50 to 60 pieces.

4. Transfer the potato pieces to a big mixing bowl then add the avocado oil tossing until well coated.

5. Add the seasoning ingredients one at a time to the potato slices, ending with nutritional yeast. Toss until well mixed before adding the next seasoning. Adjust seasonings to your taste.

6. Transfer the seasoned sweet potato slices to a parchment paper lined baking pan then bake for 15 to 20 minutes at 425°F.

7. Take out the pan from the oven then flip the fries over then return to th oven for about 5 to 10 minutes until a bit crispy and don't burn.

8. Serve hot. Enjoy!

Nutritional Information: Calories: 34kcal; Total Fat: 1.5g; Total Carb: 4.5g; Protein: 1.2g

Creamy Cauli Chocó Smoothie Bowl

Preparation time: 5 minutes

Cooking time: 0 minute

Servings: 1 - 2

Ingredients:

For the cream:

1 cup frozen organic cauliflower rice

1 large frozen organic banana

2 tbsp organic raw powdered cacao

1 tbsp organic almond butter

¼ cup plus 1 tbsp almond milk, homemade

For the toppings:

1 - 2 tbsp organic raw cacao nibs

½ cup wild blueberries, organic

Directions:

1. Pour all the cream ingredients into a blender then process on high speed until well mixed has a soft-serve ice cream texture, use the tamper if required.

2. Transfer mixture to serving bowls.

3. Top with toppings like cacao nibs and wild blueberries or desired healthy and fruit toppings. Enjoy!

Nutritional Information: Calories: 423kcal; Total Fat: 17.2g; Total Carb: 56g; Protein: 11.1g

No-Bake Cherry Black Forest Brownies

Preparation time: 10 minutes

Cooking time: 4 hours

Servings: 8 small brownies

Ingredients:

For the cherry filling:

1 tbsp organic coconut oil, refined

8 large pitted organic medjool dates

1½ cups pitted organic cherries, halved

For the brownie base:

¼ cup organic raw powdered cacao

1 cup organic walnuts

2 tbsp organic coconut oil, refined

4 organic pitted medjool dates

1 pinch of Himalayan pink salt

For the Chocó topping:

2 tbsp organic raw powdered cacao

1 organic avocado

2 tbsp organic date nectar

2 tbsp organic coconut oil, refined

2 tbsp organic almond butter

Directions:

1. Prepare the brownie base; pour all the brownie base ingredients into a blender then process until well mixed, moist and crumbly.

2. Transfer mixture to a parchment paper lined n 8 by 5" baking pan, pressing down the mixture with your hands or the back of a spoon on the bottom of the pan then set aside.

3. Prepare the cherry filling; remove the seeds by slicing the cherry in half and taking out the seed then remove stem by cutting them off. Transfer the cherries to a small bowl.

4. Pour the cherry filling ingredients into a blender then process it 10 to 12 long times, enough to crush the cherries and dates into chunks but not over processed.

5. Transfer the mixture to the baking pan then spread out over the brownie base, pressing down with your hands or the back of a spoon. Set aside.

6. Prepare the Chocó topping; combine all Chocó toppings ingredients in a small bowl then whisk until smooth, creamy and there isn't any visible pieces of avocado.

7. Pour the chocolate topping into the baking pan then spread over the cherry filling.

8. Freeze the pan in the freezer for about 3 to 4 hours until solid.

9. When ready to serve, take out from the freezer then allow it sit on the counter top for some minutes for easy slice.

10. Freeze in a BPA-free air-tight container until ready to serve. Note that it gets soft when left out room temp. Enjoy!

Nutritional Information: Calories 638kcal; Total Fat: 49g; Total Carb: 42.1g; Protein: 10.9g

Chocó Raspberry Ice Cream Bar

Preparation time: 5 minutes

Cooking time: 2 hours

Servings: 10 - 12 squares

Ingredients:

For the ice cream:

13.5 oz organic full-fat coconut milk

2 pitted organic avocados

¼ cup organic date nectar

¼ tsp Himalayan pink salt

½ cup organic raw powdered cacao

¼ tsp organic powdered vanilla bean

For the topping:

½ cup organic raspberries, freeze-dried

Other Ingredient:

1 cup organic raspberries, freeze-dried

Directions:

1. Refrigerate the can of full-fat coconut milk for 1 hour before making this recipe because you will use the fat portion and not liquid.

2. Take out the can of coconut milk from the freezer the scoop out the solidified coconut fat portion into a blender. Reserve the coconut liquid for a smoothie.

3. Pour all the rest of the ice cream ingredients into the blender then process until smooth and creamy.

4. Pour in 1 cup of the freeze-dried raspberries then stir gently by hand, don't blend them.

5. Transfer mixture to a parchment paper lined 8 by 5" bread pan then spread out evenly in the pan.

6. Add ½ cup freeze-dried raspberries on top of the ice cream mixture then freeze for about 2 to 3 hours or solid.

7. Once ready to serve, take out from the freezer then slice into small squares or rectangle bars.

8. Freeze in a BPA-free air-tight container until ready to serve. Note that they get soft when left out at room temp. Enjoy!

Nutritional Information: Calories: 231kcal; Total Fat: 17.9g; Total Carb: 14.2g; Protein: 1.7g

Chocó Coated Strawberry Truffles

Preparation time: 5 minutes

Cooking time: 30 minutes

Servings: 10 - 12 small truffles

Ingredients:

For the Chocó coating:

1 tsp organic coconut oil

½ cup cacao dark chocolate morsels

For the truffles:

8 pitted large organic medjool dates

2 cups organic freeze-dried strawberries

Directions:

1. Prepare the truffles; combine all the truffles ingredients in a blender then process until crumbly and sticky.

2. Scoop out a small spoonful then mold into ball shape then set aside.

3. Prepare the chocolate coating by combining all the coating ingredients in a small sauce pan then melt on very low heat, stirring until smooth.

4. To assemble; place each truffle ball in the saucepan with the melted chocolate then toss around gently until completely coated.

5. Take out from the saucepan then transfer to a parchment paper lined baking pan or plate.

6. Freeze for about 15 to 30 minutes until solid.

7. Refrigerate or freeze in a BPA-free air-tight container until ready to serve. Note that it becomes soft when left out at room temp. Enjoy!

Nutritional Information: Calories: 352kcal; Total Fat: 2.3g; Total Carb: 86.1g; Protein: 0.5g

Cheesy Baked Mushrooms

Preparation time: 5 minutes

Cooking time: 20 minutes

Servings: 1 - 2

Ingredients:

2 cups organic baby bella mushrooms, stem removed then sliced

1 cup almond milk, homemade

For the seasoning:

½ cup nutritional yeast

½ cup almond flour

½ tsp organic ground powdered garlic

¼ - ½ tsp organic ground cayenne pepper

½ tsp Himalayan pink salt

Directions:

1. Preheat the oven to 425°F.

2. Prepare the seasoning by combining all the seasoning ingredients in a small bowl then stir until well mixed. Adjust seasonings like garlic, pepper and salt to your taste. Use ¼ tsp or less of cayenne pepper for less spicy then set aside.

3. Remove mushroom stem then slice and set aside.

4. To assemble; get a small bowl of mushroom slices, a small bowl of almond milk, a small bowl containing ½ of the seasoning mix and a parchment paper lined baking pan.

5. Coat the mushroom slices in the bowl of milk until well coated.

6. Take out the mushrooms with a fork, allowing excess milk drip off then dredge them in the bowl of seasoning. Toss again until well coated.

7. Transfer them to the prepared baking pan then spread out gently so they don't overlap or over each other.

8. Repeat coating process with the other cup of mushrooms, making use the same bowl of milk, and the other ½ of the seasoning mix.

9. Bake for 10 minutes at 425°F.

10. Remove from the oven then flip the mushrooms over to bake the other side.

11. Return to the oven and bake for another 10 minutes.

12. Take out from the oven and serve hot. Enjoy!

Nutritional Information: Calories: 255kcal; Total Fat: 7.7g; Total Carb: 29.2g; Protein: 25.6g

Chocó Vanilla Pistachio Fudge Cups

Preparation time: 5 minutes

Cooking time: 60 minutes

Servings: 24 mini cups

Ingredients:

¼ cup organic raw powdered cacao

1 cup chopped organic pistachios

1 tsp organic powdered vanilla bean

¼ cup organic date nectar

1 cup melted organic coconut oil

¼ cup organic almond butter

For the topping: Sea salt

Directions:

1. Combine all the ingredients in a medium-sized bowl then stir until smooth and well mixed.

2. Scoop mixture into 24 mini-muffin cups.

3. Set the mini-muffin cups on a baking sheet then freeze for about 5 to 10 minutes or long enough for the surface to solidify a bit.

4. Take out the baking sheet from the freezer then sprinkle with sea salt. Note that if the fudge top isn't solid, the salt will sink in.

5. Return the baking pan to the freezer for about 30 to 60 minutes until solid.

6. Refrigerate or freeze in a BPA-free air-tight container until ready to serve. Note that they will become soft when left out at room temp. Enjoy!

Nutritional Information: Calories: 196kcal; Total Fat: 21.1g; Total Carb: 2.4g; Protein: 1.1g

Cheesy Broccoli Bites

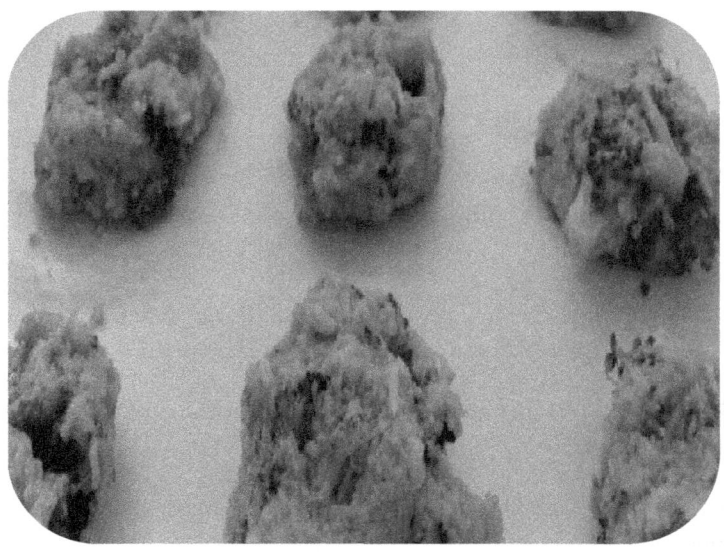

Preparation time: 5 minutes

Cooking time: 20 minutes

Servings: 3 cups

Ingredients:

For the broccoli:

2 tablespoons 100% pure avocado oil

3 cups organic broccoli florets

For the seasoning:

¼ cup nutritional yeast

¼ cup almond flour

1/8 - ¼ tsp organic ground cayenne pepper

¼ tsp organic ground powdered garlic

¼ tsp Himalayan pink salt

Directions:

1. Preheat the oven to 400°F.

2. Prepare the seasoning by combining all the seasoning ingredients in a small bowl then stir until well mixed. Adjust seasonings to your taste then set aside.

3. Prepare the broccoli; pour the broccoli florets into a large bowl then ladle avocado oil on top. Toss together until well coated.

4. Sprinkle ½ of the seasoning mix over broccoli pieces then toss gently until well coated.

5. Set the seasoned broccoli pieces on a parchment paper lined baking pan then bake for 10 minutes at 400°F.

6. Take out the pan from the oven then transfer the broccoli pieces to the large bowl.

7. Sprinkle the remaining ½ of the seasoning mix over the baked broccoli then toss again gently until well coated.

8. Return to the baking pan then to the oven and bake for another 20 to 25 minutes, or until crispy. Enjoy!

Nutritional Information: Calories: 155kcal; Total Fat: 10.8g; Total Carb: 9.4g; Protein: 7.1g

Lectin-Free Chocó Avocado Frosting

Preparation time: 5 minutes

Cooking time: 0 minute

Servings: 1 cup

Ingredients:

¼ cup organic raw powdered cacao

2 organic avocados

¼ cup organic date nectar/ organic coconut nectar or maple syrup

¼ cup organic almond butter

1 - 2 pinches of Himalayan pink salt

Directions:

1. Combine avocados and the remaining ingredients in a small bowl until thick, smooth, creamy and without any pieces.

2. Refrigerate for about 15 to 30 minutes for thicker frosting and to thicker it. Enjoy!

Nutritional Information: Calories: 392kcal; Total Fat: 30.3g; Total Carb: 28.1g; Protein: 4g

The End

CPSIA information can be obtained
at www.ICGtesting.com
Printed in the USA
LVHW102154120822
725822LV00004B/210